# Non-medical Prescribing

# Non-medical Prescribing

**Edited by**

**Mahesh Sodha** BSc(Hons), DipClinPharm, MSc, FRPharmS

Community pharmacist, Essex, and Visiting Fellow at the School of Pharmacy, University of Hertfordshire, UK

and

**Soraya Dhillon** MBE, BPharm, PhD, FRPharmS

Foundation Professor and Head of The School of Pharmacy at the University of Hertfordshire, UK

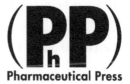

**Pharmaceutical Press**

Published by the Pharmaceutical Press
**An imprint of RPS Publishing**

66-68 East Smithfield, London E1W 1AW, UK

(**PP**) is a trade mark of RPS Publishing
RPS Publishing is the publishing organisation of the Royal Pharmaceutical Society
of Great Britain

First published 2009

Typeset by J&L Composition, Scarborough, North Yorkshire
Printed in Great Britain by TJ International Ltd, Padstow, Cornwall

ISBN 978 0 85369 768 8

A catalogue record for this book is available from the British Library.

# Contents

# Preface

This book has been designed to serve as a resource for all non-medical prescribers and will be particularly useful to nurses, pharmacists, optometrists, physiotherapists and other healthcare professionals who desire to become supplementary or independent prescribers in their field.

While we have attempted to make the book comprehensive, it is not intended to be an exhaustive text on the subject and the reader is referred to other sources for more detailed information in areas such as consultation skills.

The book provides an overview of key areas which consider safe and effective prescribing. The second part provides clinical topics, with prescriber insights and reflections and clinical case studies for support.

The authors direct readers to other reference sources to expand understanding, knowledge and skills in core clinical areas.

The book is a useful resource for undergraduate pharmacy, nursing and medical prescribers as well as health practitioners who intend to become independent prescribers.

# About the Editors

## Mahesh Sodha

Mahesh Sodha is a community pharmacist with a practice in Chelmsford, Essex, and a visiting fellow at the School of Pharmacy, University of Hertfordshire. He has extensive experience of both primary and secondary care and has a special interest in oncology, palliative care and diabetes. He has worked part time as a practice research pharmacist and published research in the areas of nurse prescribing, GP practice work and palliative care. Mahesh has also worked as a cancer lead and served as a member of the professional executive committee and board of a Primary Care Trust. He currently practises as an independent prescribing pharmacist and runs clinics managing patients with diabetes, hypertension, dyslipidaemia and chronic kidney disease.

In June 2005, Mahesh was designated as a Fellow of the Royal Pharmaceutical Society of Great Britain for attaining distinction in the practice and profession of pharmacy.

## Soraya Dhillon

Soraya Dhillon is a foundation professor and head of the School of Pharmacy at the University of Hertfordshire. Professor Dhillon has extensive experience in clinical pharmacy and clinical pharmacokinetics and has held positions in community and hospital pharmacy. She is published widely in the evaluation of clinical pharmacy services and education. Her career has involved her developing and evaluating clinical service. Her work has supported the development of a postgraduate education framework for pharmacists in hospital and community. In her current role she has developed an undergraduate MPharm degree which has been built on the principles of vertical and horizontal integration of the science to underpin evidence-based practice. The undergraduate degree also incorporates prescribing modules at Level 3 and M to provide new graduates with the underpinning knowledge and skills to then pursue non-medical prescribing courses following graduation. She currently holds a non-executive role as chairman of Luton & Dunstable Foundation Trust and has a particular interest in driving forward patient safety initiatives.

# Contributors

**Dr Kiren Gill**  BSc, MBBS, DRCOG
Specialist trainee in obstetrics and gynaecology at Whittington Hospital, London
Visiting Fellow, School of Pharmacy, University of Hertfordshire

**Jo Noble-Gresty**  BPharm(Hons), MRPharmS, SP, IP, Certificate in Pharmacy Practice, MSc in Pain Management
Member of the Palliative Care Pharmacists Network
Steering group member of the Independent Teaching Group for Palliative Medicine

**Dr Andrzej Kostrzewski**  MSc, MMedEd, MRPharmS, FHEA
Academic Manager in Clinical Pharmacy, School of Pharmacy, University of Hertfordshire

**Dr Richard O'Neill**  LLB, LLM, BPharm, PhD, MRPharmS
Associate Head of School, School of Pharmacy, University of Hertfordshire

**Dr Maxine Offredy**  BA(Hons), PhD
Reader in Primary Health Care, Centre for Research in Primary and Community Care, University of Hertfordshire

**Professor Fabrizio Schifano**  MD, MRCPsych, Dip Clin Pharmacology, Dip Psychiatry
Chair in Clinical Pharmacology and Therapeutics
Associate Dean, Postgraduate Medical School
Hon Consultant Psychiatrist (Addictions), University of Hertfordshire

**Nader Siabi**  BSc, MSc, SP, IP, MRPharmS
Senior Clinical Practitioner, School of Pharmacy, University of Hertfordshire

**Professor Alan Sinclair** BSc, MBBS, MRCP, MD, MSc, FRCP
Professor of Medicine and Consultant Diabetologist, Beds & Herts
Postgraduate Medical School, University of Hertfordshire

**Dr Nicola Stoner** BSc(Hons), MRPharmS (SPresc & IPresc), DipClinPharm,
PhD, ACPP(FCP), RICR
Honorary Principal Visiting Fellow, The School of Pharmacy, The University
of Reading
Consultant Pharmacist – Cancer, Oxford Cancer Centre and Cancer Research
UK, Oxford Radcliffe Hospital

**Helen Williams** BPharm(Hons), MRPharmS (IPresc), PGDip(Cardiol)
Consultant Pharmacist for Cardiovascular Disease, South East London
NHS Lambeth, Southwark Health and Social Care and South London
Cardiac and Stroke Networks

**Professor Joy Wingfield** LLM, MPhil, BPharm, DipAgVetPharm,
FRPharmS, MCPP
Special Professor of Pharmacy Law and Ethics, University of Nottingham
Visiting Professor, School of Pharmacy, University of Hertfordshire

# 1

# Development of non-medical prescribing – Historical background and competency framework for successful prescribing

*Maxine Offredy*

---

**Key learning points:**

- Understand the importance of non-medical prescribing and its historical developments
- Understand the principles of competency
- Understand the necessity for competency frameworks
- Describe the importance of issues relating to successful prescribing.

---

## Introduction

This chapter provides an outline of the historical development of non-medical prescribing, before taking the reader through a discussion of competency, competency framework and issues relating to successful prescribing. The discussion is placed within the context of the current healthcare climate.

The concept of non-medical prescribing in England has its genesis in the Cumberlege Report (Department of Health and Social Security, 1986), which suggested that community nurses should be able to prescribe some medication as part of their routine care for patients. A similar suggestion was made 3 years later in the Crown Report (Department of Health, 1989), pointing to the potential benefits of patient care, better use of patients', nurses' and GPs' time and clearer lines of responsibility. These suggestions continue to be a platform for the current UK government's drive to increase and improve patients' access to healthcare. The recommendations led to legislation being passed in 1992, and in 1994 nurses in eight demonstration sites were permitted to prescribe from a limited formulary. The success of the demonstration sites paved the way for district nurses and health visitors (or practice nurses with a district nurse or health visitor qualification) in England to prescribe from a limited formulary. However, issues such as funding, legal technicalities and the medical profession's reluctance to extend prescribing rights to nurses had to be addressed before nurse prescribing became a national policy (Campbell and Collins, 2001).

The introduction of a new Labour administration in 1997 accelerated the pace of change for nurse/non-medical prescribing policies and in 2000 the Department of Health endorsed earlier recommendations for nurses and professions allied to medicine to prescribe some drugs. A drawback to this accelerated change of pace is that the research literature on non-medical prescribing has not kept pace with policy changes. The literature available on nurse prescribing is largely descriptive and relatively small scale, and few publications address the context, process and complexities of nurse prescribing (Offredy *et al.*, 2008).

A further introduction of policy changes for non-medical prescribing was established in May 2006, whereby nurses and pharmacists gained extended prescribing powers. From May 2006, qualified nurse prescribers are now able to prescribe any licensed medicine for any medical condition within their competence, including some controlled drugs which can be prescribed independently for specific conditions only. Once qualified, pharmacist independent prescribers will be able to prescribe any licensed medicine for any medical condition within their competence, with the exception of controlled drugs. The purpose of the government's non-medical prescribing programme is threefold: to give patients quicker access to medicines; to improve access to services, and to make better use of nurses' and other health professionals' skills. This extension of prescribing powers was not without its critics. Doctors' leaders said the decision was 'irresponsible and dangerous' (Miller, 2005). However, Pruce (2005) of the Royal Pharmaceutical Society of Great Britain saw the move as a 'significant milestone which would benefit patients'.

In addition to independent prescribing by nurses and pharmacists, supplementary prescribing enables qualified nurses and pharmacists to prescribe any medicine (including controlled drugs) within the framework of a patient-specific clinical management plan, agreed with a doctor and the patient. Supplementary prescribing will remain an option for nurse and pharmacist prescribers, particularly in complex areas of prescribing such as mental health or situations in which prescribers need to consolidate their experience.

Since April 2005, physiotherapists, chiropodists/podiatrists and radiographers have also been able to qualify as supplementary prescribers. Changes to regulations to enable optometrists to train and register as supplementary prescribers came into force in July 2005. It is the government's intention that optometrists who wish to take on independent prescribing responsibilities will have the opportunity to undertake training provided by a Higher Education Institution and accredited by the General Optical Council (GOC). Once trained, optometrists will be able to prescribe any licensed medicine for ocular conditions affecting the eye and the tissues surrounding the eye within the recognised area of expertise and competence of the optometrist. To date, the government envisage that medicines for non-ocular conditions and controlled drugs will not be prescribable by optometrists. As with other non-medical prescribers, optometrists will have to undertake continuing education and training to keep their skills up-to-date and maintain their specialty registration as a prescriber with the GOC. The proposed changes are applicable throughout the UK in the NHS, the independent and voluntary sectors. Further, since 2007 qualified nurses who do not hold a specialist practitioner qualification may prescribe from the Community Nurses Prescriber's Formulary, following educational preparation laid down by the Nursing and Midwifery Council.

Thus, a wide range of healthcare professionals are able to prescribe medicines for their patients, giving quicker access to treatment and healthcare and fulfilling the original goals of non-medical prescribing set out more than 20 years ago. Nonetheless, to be able to prescribe one must be competent to do so. The next section addresses the issue of competency, followed by a discussion on competency frameworks.

## Competency

The movement towards what is now established practice of addressing competence of individuals in the workplace emerged in the 1980s after the publication of Richard Boyatzis' (1982) book, *The Competent Manager: A model for effective performance*, about competent people. The concept has been influential in many areas of work life and is now widely used in, and accepted by, human resources departments of organisations as an essential quality for employees to possess. Professional discourse during the 1980s and 1990s centred on whether the term should be 'competency' or 'competence', but nowadays both terms are used interchangeably. Thus, currently there is no single definition of the concepts as exemplified below.

Boyatzis (1982) sees competency as:

*an underlying characteristic of a person which results in effective action and/or superior performance in a job* while Kak *et al.* (2001) define competency as:

> *the ability of a health worker to perform according to predefined standards. Competency is developed through pre-service education, in-service training, hands-on experience, and the assistance of mentors and preceptors.*

Roach (1992) takes a different view of competence:

> *the state of having the knowledge, judgement, skills, energy, experience and motivation required to respond adequately to the demands of one's professional responsibilities.*

Both the UK Training Agency (1988) and Fletcher (1991) emphasise the ability to perform activities within an occupation as key to the definition of competence. The common theme in the above definitions is that competency/competence is a personal attribute. However, Stuart (1989) sees competence as being external and independent of the individual and opines that:

> *While an individual may be deemed 'competent,' 'occupational competence' relates to the functions associated with an occupation. Standards of competence are used to describe the characteristics of the functions and so are independent of the individual.*

What is clear from these definitions is that competence is a dynamic function that can be applied to a professional individual at any stage in their career because the contexts within which health professionals operate and the concomitant demands being placed upon them are subject to continual change. Thus, standards will take account of changes in practice and will vary with experience and expectations. These definitions of competency/competence include words such as knowledge, skills, attitudes and experience. Competence can therefore be seen as a combination of these which contribute to the standards required for successful job performance. For example, making the correct prescribing decisions are the result of combining key activities of knowledge, skills, attitudes and experience to reach that decision. Therefore, competence must be contextualised to the requirement of the service and/or organisation and will differ widely according to the user's objectives.

Having discussed some of the issues associated with defining competencies, we now turn to discussing competency framework and its uses.

## Competency framework

A competency framework is a set of competencies or behaviours that are important for successful performance; it seeks to address the needs of decision makers in organisations. It also provides organisations with a common language to describe a set of characteristics or qualities that are required for performance. Development of competencies should help individuals to continually improve their performance and to work more effectively (NPC Plus, 2007). Thus, they define the how of delivery and are used in a number of situations such as: recruitment and selection; training and development; probationary period; performance review and promoting equality and diversity (Department of Health, 2004).

Established frameworks for prescribing include those for:

- pharmacists
- optometrists
- chiropodists/podiatrists
- physiotherapists
- radiographers and
- nurses (Department of Health, 2005).

In general, competency frameworks for the above professionals have a similar format but the details will differ according to the requirements of the profession. The discipline of pharmacy will be used as an example. The competency framework for pharmacist prescribers has three main areas of competency: (1) the consultation; (2) effective prescribing; and (3) contextual prescribing. These three areas are further broken down into three competencies, giving a total of nine competencies. Each of the nine competencies has an overarching statement indicating what the competency is about. The overarching statement is further broken down into specific behavioural indicators which provide details of actions that would be demonstrated if the competency is undertaken effectively. *Figure 1.1* shows the breakdown of the competence area of the consultation.

Healthcare providers such as pharmacists, optometrists, nurses and doctors must demonstrate that they are competent to provide care by achieving the minimum standard of competence in their training. Once trained, Kak *et al.* (2001) say that healthcare organisations should continually measure competence and gives 10 reasons for doing so. These are explained next.

## Reasons for measuring competence in healthcare

### Changes in healthcare

Continual changes in healthcare policies provide the impetus for policy makers to put in place access to continuing training for their employees to ensure competence in the workplace.

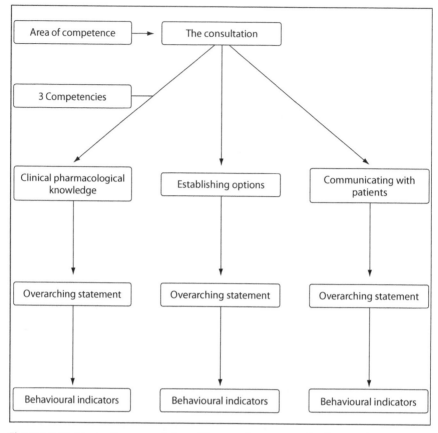

**Figure 1.1** Diagrammatic representation of the area of competence for the consultation process in the pharmacy competency framework.

### Assessing individual performance

Competency assessment can play an important role in an organisation's performance improvement initiatives by focusing on individual providers or groups of providers where gaps have been identified.

### Selection of new staff

Competency assessment is useful when recruiting new staff to ensure they can do the job they are hired to do or could do it with reasonable orientation/training.

## Organisational performance

Assessments of organisational performance need to be undertaken to ascertain the effectiveness of services provided. The results assist organisations in deciding whether or not training needs to be redesigned.

## Liability

Healthcare organisations are responsible for the quality of care their staff provide and consequently must ensure that staff are competent and can meet standards for the provision of care. Assessing providers' competence periodically enables healthcare organisations to meet this crucial responsibility.

## Risk management

Competency assessments can be used to monitor employees' knowledge of the organisation's policies and procedures, particularly in high-risk areas. Feedback from these assessments can be implemented in future training and continuing education in endeavouring to improve overall performance.

## Certification/approval of providers

Competency assessment forms an integral part of the certification and/or approval processes of service providers. For example, in England and Wales, the Healthcare Commission are responsible for assessing and reporting on the performance of both the NHS and independent healthcare organisations to ensure that they continue to provide a high standard of care (Healthcare Commission, 2005). Investors in People, on the other hand, is an internationally recognised quality standard for the development of organisations through good workforce development practice. It provides a framework for improving organisational performance through a planned approach (Investors in People, 2001).

## Measuring training outcomes

Competency assessments may be used to ascertain the effectiveness of training in closing the knowledge–skills gap. Low scores on competence assessments after training may be an indication that the training was ineffective, poorly designed, poorly presented or inappropriate. Trainers can use this information to improve training content or delivery.

### Planning for new services

Competency assessment can help managers identify providers who are competent to provide a new clinical service, providers who need improvements in specific knowledge or skill areas when a new service is offered, and providers who are ready to act as mentors of newly trained providers. It can also be used to inform the commissioning process.

### Supervision

Competency assessments can guide healthcare managers in providing performance improvement feedback to healthcare providers.

Thus, frameworks can be used in a variety of situations to assist both individuals and organisations in the quest to achieve effective healthcare. It can take a broader vision and a more pragmatic approach that can incorporate practitioners' personal attributes to make healthcare processes more effective. Another dimension of the effective healthcare paradigm is that of successful prescribing, which forms the discussion of the next section.

## Successful prescribing

Successful prescribing depends on a number of interrelated factors, such as providing information that is tailored, clear, accurate and in sufficient detail to aid understanding by the patient. A repeated finding in the international literature is that patients prefer health professionals who listen and encourage them to discuss their problems (Grol *et al.*, 1999; Richards, 1999). As prescriptions will now be written in places other than general practice, it is important that there is effective communication between prescriber and patient given the continuing problem of non-adherence to treatment and patients' priorities for prescribing (Royal Pharmaceutical Society, 1997).

In 2002, the Department of Health supported recommendations by the Royal Pharmaceutical Society to use the term 'concordance' when referring to the process of prescribing and medicine taking. Concordance is defined by Medicines Partnership as a 'new way to define the process of successful prescribing and medicine taking, based on partnership' (www.medicines-partnership.org/about-us/concordance). The model for concordance shares a similar format to the framework structure outlined above in Figure 1.1. The concordant framework has three main components: (1) patients have enough knowledge to participate as partners; (2) prescribing consultations involve patients as partners and (3) patients are supported in taking medicines. Each of these three components has associated indicators which, if implemented, fulfil the criteria for the components, thus leading to successful prescribing. Shared decision making, which is the essence of concordance, has its own competency framework (NPC Plus, 2007) based on the format outlined above for health professionals and represented in Figure 1.1.

However, criticisms have been levelled at the concordance model. Heath (2003) argues that proponents of the model place undue emphasis on health professionals' failures to establish therapeutic partnerships with their patients despite the paucity of evidence to show the correlation between (1) improved patient information and increased medicine taking behaviour and (2) the effectiveness of more training and education of healthcare professionals to endeavour to improve patients' behaviour in taking medication. She argues that the professional literature ignores issues relating to diverse clinical circumstances, such as conditions that could affect the community or those that could affect the individual. In terms of health education literature for patients, Heath (2003) points to the lack of discussion on topics such as numbers needed to treat and numbers needed to harm. She argues that this information is needed in the patient literature so that they are cognisant of both benefits and harms of drugs and are helped to make decisions based on this information as well as their own valuation of possible outcomes. However, Lewis *et al.* (2003) found that patients and health professionals find the concepts of risk and benefit difficult to understand and doctors were more likely to accept fewer benefits than their patients when deciding whether to start preventative treatment.

Macfarlane *et al.* (1997) support the view that healthcare outcomes tend to be better when patients are informed and supported to participate in decisions because there is a higher rate of patient satisfaction and services are used more appropriately. Studies also show that patients and professionals have different ideas about good-quality care (Jung *et al.*, 1997) and arguably this includes prescribing. Safe and effective prescribing must be the core competency to be expected of medical and non-medical prescribers, who must demonstrate a firm grasp of pharmacology and therapeutics. Studies have shown that some groups of non-medical prescribers require further training and education in pharmacology to support their role as non-medical prescribers (Sodha *et al.*, 2002; Offredy *et al.*, 2008). These skills are particularly important when consideration is given to the prescribing privileges of independent non-medical prescribers; pharmaceutical developments that indicate new ways of prescribing; complexity of drug use; increasing use of litigation; focus on the elderly and chronically ill who are more likely to be on more than three types of medication and who are more prone to adverse effects of drugs (Leathard *et al.*, 2006). Given that many non-medical prescribers may lack the necessary chemistry background that would be desirable for a pharmacology degree, Leathard *et al.* (2006: 8) posit that:

*The content of any course needs ... to be based on taking a prag-
matic view of the need to meet students where they are: making
creative use of analogies and images to illustrate pharmacological
principles ... and building on the wealth of experience of
prescribing students ... while expecting little in the way of
bioscience background knowledge.*

Multifaceted interventions can lead to successful prescribing. The interventions include combining patient education in a variety of venues and
formats; structured, practical interactive tutorials that involve the application
of pharmacological knowledge in clinical scenarios (Sodha *et al.*, 2002);
prescriber characteristics and prescribing policies. Prescribing policies require
an active commitment from the prescriber, adequate feedback from the
reviewer and positive reinforcement. A key challenge for those new to patient
examination is to develop the required skills along with expertise in interpreting findings. Monitoring patients' responses to therapy and identifying
adverse effects are also important. In some cases, the non-medical prescriber
may need to work with multidisciplinary teams as well as maintaining
competency by in-service training or other types of update programmes.

## Summary

We have seen that the drive for non-medical prescribing had a slow
beginning but has progressed quickly since the late 1990s, and currently
involves a wide range of health professionals. This move is to be welcomed.
However, healthcare professionals must ensure that they are competent to
perform their role. Information about medicines for patients must also be in
a format that recognises their preferences and values.

## References

Boyatzis R E (1982). *The Competent Manager: A model for effective performance*. London:
    Wiley.
Campbell P and Collins G (2001). Prescribing for community nurses. *Nurs Times* 97: 38–39.
Department of Health (1989). *Review of Prescribing, Supply and Administration of Medicines
    (The Crown Report)*. London: Department of Health.
Department of Health (2000). *The NHS Plan: A plan for investment, a plan for reform*.
    London: The Stationery Office.
Department of Health (2004). *The NHS Knowledge and Skills Framework (NHS KSF) and the
    Development Review Process*. London: Department of Health.
Department of Health (2005). *Supplementary Prescribing by Nurses, Pharmacists,
    Chiropodists/podiatrists, Physiotherapists and Radiographers within the NHS in England*.
    London: Department of Health.
Department of Health and Social Security (1986). *Neighbourhood Nursing: A focus for care.
    Report of the Community Nursing Review*. London: HMSO.
Fletcher S (1991). *Standards and Competence: A practical guide for employers, managers and
    trainers*. London: Kogan Page.

Grol R, Wensing M, Mainz J, Ferreira P and Hearnshaw H (1999). Patients' priorities with respect to general practice care: an international comparison. *Fam Pract* 16: 4–11.

Healthcare Commission (2005). *Assessment for Improvement: The annual health check – measuring what matters*. London: Healthcare Commission.

Heath I (2003). A wolf in sheep's clothing: a critical look at the ethics of drug taking. *BMJ* 327: 856–858.

Investors in People UK (2001). *A Decade of Success:10 years of making a difference to working life in the UK*. London: Investors in People UK.

Jung H, Wensing M and Grol R (1997). What makes a good general practitioner: do patients and doctors have different views? *Br J Gen Pract* 47: 805–809.

Kak N, Burkhalter B and Cooper M (2001). Measuring the competence of healthcare providers. *Qual Assur* 2: 1–28.

Leathard H L, Abbott M, Brownsell M, Lennard M and Maxwell S (2006). Education for new prescribers: a summary of proceedings of a symposium held at the British Pharmaceutical Society, December 2005. *Br J Pharmacol* 63: 5–9.

Lewis D K, Robinson J and Wilkinson F (2003). Factors involved in deciding to start preventative treatment: qualitative study of clinicians' and lay people's attitudes. *BMJ* 327: 822–823.

Macfarlane J T, Holmes W F and Macfarlane R M (1997). Reducing reconsultations for acute lower respiratory tract illness with an information leaflet: a randomised controlled study of patients in primary care. *Br J Gen Pract* 47: 719–722.

Miller P (2005). Nurse prescribing plans opposed. BBC News. http:www.news.bbc.co.uk/1/hi/health/4424112.stm (accessed 5 August 2007).

NPC Plus (2007). *Maintaining Competency in Prescribing: An outline to help pharmacist prescribers*. Keele: Keele University Science and Business Park.

Offredy M, Kendall S and Goodman C (2008). The use of cognitive continuum theory and patient scenarios to explore nurse prescribers' pharmacological knowledge and decision-making. *Int J Nurs Stud* 45: 855–868.

Pruce D (2005). Nurse prescribing plans opposed. BBC News. http:www.news.bbc.co.uk/1/hi/health/4424112.stm (accessed 5 August 2007).

Richards T (1999). Patients' priorities. *BMJ* 318: 277.

Roach S (1992). *The Human Act of Caring: A blueprint for the health professions* (revised edition). Ottawa: Canadian Hospital Association Press.

Royal Pharmaceutical Society (1997). *From Compliance to Concordance: Towards shared goals in medicine taking*. London: Royal Pharmaceutical Society.

Sodha M, Williams G, Shah R and Clegg J (2002). Nurse prescribing: testing the knowledge base. *J Community Nurs* 16: 4–14.

Stuart D (1989). The concept of occupational competence. *Competence Assessment* 8: 11.

UK Training Agency (1988). The development of assessable standards for national certification. Guidance note 1 – a code of practice and a development model. Training Agency, Sheffield.

# 2

# Legal and ethical aspects of prescribing

*Joy Wingfield*

---

**Key learning points:**

- Your liability for harmful effects of prescribing is affected by whether a medicine is licensed, is used outside of its licence or is unlicensed

- There are four legal categories of medicines: controlled drugs (CDs), prescription only medicines (POMs), pharmacy only (P) medicines and General Sale List (GSL) medicines

- The law specifies who can become independent and supplementary prescribers, what they can prescribe and under what circumstances and what must appear on a prescription

- Non-medical prescribers should be aware of how medicines may be supplied other than on prescription, in particular through the use of patient group directions (PGDs)

- Non-medical prescribers should take care to seek consent to their interventions and to respect the confidential nature of their prescribing information.

---

## Introduction

Perhaps the first thing to note is that the law generally makes no distinction between healthcare provided within the National Health Service (NHS) and that provided elsewhere, in the private or voluntary sectors. The law controlling the supply of medicines applies within hospitals, clinics, GP surgeries, care homes, pharmacies, newsagents and even supplies to a patient in his of her own home. A few readers may remember something called 'Crown Immunity' which provided exemption from the law and greater latitude over supplies of medicines within hospitals because they were (originally) owned by the State; this exemption was formally removed from NHS hospitals in April 1991. Moreover, the concept of Crown Immunity is now no longer applicable to health services in prisons and the armed forces; all are expected to meet the same standards of quality and clinical governance (other than in exceptional cases).

However, administrative law (see below), which underpins the structures and operation of the NHS, now does vary significantly between the home countries of England, Scotland, Wales and Northern Ireland, although the broad principles remain very similar. Finally, all health professionals and those who work with them to deliver healthcare should behave ethically. Most health professions will have a published Code of Ethics or other Code of Practice or Standards that sets out the values, attitudes and behaviours expected of them in their practice. The wording may differ but the sentiments will be consistent.

## The law relating to prescribing

'The law' is a very wide topic. We should first of all distinguish between several types of law; the distinctions are important because they dictate the nature of the sanction if you break the law! The form of law familiar to most of us is statutory criminal law – the stuff of television shows and films with police and criminals (and lawyers and courts) locked in perpetual contests. Statutory law comprises one of two main divisions of law: statute law and civil law. A statute is, strictly speaking, an Act of Parliament. In the context of prescribing, the two Acts you should be familiar with are the Medicines Act 1968 and the Misuse of Drugs Act 1971. We cover them in detail below. All Acts have to be put before Parliament (in the name of the Queen) where they are debated and amended and eventually emerge as an Act. An Act constitutes the 'bones' of a body of law; the 'flesh' is then added in the form of Statutory Instruments such as Regulations and Orders, which provide the detail of how the Act will be implemented. Acts are usually termed 'primary' legislation; Statutory Instruments are called 'secondary' legislation. The whole body of law, primary and secondary, is called statutory law.

Statutory law can then be characterised by the penalty for breach of the law. The most familiar to us is statutory criminal law. Breaking and entering a house can result in prison or a fine if you are caught. Breach of the Medicines Act similarly attracts criminal sanctions such as fines or prison. Almost all health professionals are now regulated by a regulatory authority such as the Nursing and Midwifery Council or the General Medical Council. Such bodies will have legal powers, developed and approved by Parliament, set out in statutes. The sanctions for breach of this statutory professional law may not be fines or prison but are more likely to be orders for supervised practice, suspension or removal from a professional register.

The other form of statutory law relevant to prescribers is called statutory administrative law. Every body that carries out public services – be it an ambulance trust, a primary care organisation, a hospital or your local education authority or borough council, has its powers set out in statute. Law is needed to give the public body the right, for example, to manage property, employ staff and pay them and to contract for services. Limits are also set on these powers. A public body may be held to account if it acts unfairly or exceeds its powers and this is done through the process of judicial review. Conversely a public body needs to hold those who work for it or contract with it accountable for the services they provide on its behalf, usually through tribunals rather than the criminal courts. The sanctions for breach of this kind of statutory law could be through internal disciplinary processes, loss of job or the contract or in some case fines that are paid to the public body rather than the State.

Breach of the statutory law relating to prescribing therefore could put you at risk of criminal sanctions, such as a fine or a prison sentence; could jeopardise your professional registration or could result in a challenge to your employing body or jeopardy to your job.

Before going on to provide information and strategies (in Chapter 3) to avoid these risks, we should consider the other major branch of law: the civil law. This term derives from the notion of duties and responsibilities owed between citizens to each other. The civil law has developed through court judgements based on the 'common law' – a scheme of justice in the original Courts presided over by the King in the Middle Ages to adjudicate in baronial disputes and the like, extended to create a system of common justice for all citizens. Action under civil law (a suit or being sued) allows an aggrieved party to sue for compensation from another citizen who is alleged to have 'wronged' him or her. In healthcare terms, the action is likely to be for clinical negligence in that the provider of the health service did not exercise the proper duty of care and hence caused harm to the patient.

## The Medicines Act 1968 and the Misuse of Drugs Act 1971

Readers who are pharmacists may wish to look away now since their undergraduate training and daily practice generally means they are very familiar indeed with the statutory criminal law controlling the marketing and supply of medicines. As the final suppliers, it is they who are most at risk of prosecution should this law be broken. However all prescribers should be aware of the legislation covering the commodities they are prescribing for others, and even pharmacists may welcome an update on the legal framework for non-medical prescribing. The Medicines Act has two main purposes: to assure the quality, safety and efficacy of medicines that are marketed in the UK and to maintain the safety of the public by controlling routes of access to potentially dangerous commodities like medicines. The Misuse of Drugs Act and its subordinate legislation adds an additional layer of tougher supply controls for a number of medicines with a high potential for abuse – the so-called controlled drugs. We look first at the licensing process which applies to all medicines, including controlled drugs.

## Medicinal products and the licensing system

Before the 1960s, the public were protected from harm from poisons, but the Poisons List was merely an inventory of substances known to be poisonous (Appelbe and Wingfield, 2005). Many poisons of low toxicity were included in medicines and the public was merely informed of their presence. The thalidomide tragedy in 1961 precipitated a demand for legislation to define precisely what is a medicine, as opposed to a poison, and to control the safety, quality and efficacy of medicines (the law calls them 'medicinal products') marketed in the UK. Under the Medicines Act, the definition of a medicinal product is broadly speaking something that is marketed for a 'medicinal purpose'. Thus a medicinal product is (paraphrased):

> *Any substance or combination of substances marketed for the purpose of treating or preventing disease or administration with a view to making a medical diagnosis or to restoring, correcting or modifying physiological functions. (Medicines Act 1968)*

Claims that a substance or product is a medicine will depend upon whether medicinal claims are made for it. A product that claims to be an antibiotic or for management of high blood pressure, for example, will always be considered to be a medicine. There are several fuzzy borderlines, however, such as homeopathic remedies that avoid the need for licensing by making no medicinal claims, or nutritional supplements that claim to be foods, or anti-wrinkle creams that stick to 'cosmetic' claims only – 'reduces the appearance of wrinkles'. For our purposes we shall consider the licensing process for the vast majority of medicines that you may wish to prescribe.

Before a medicinal product can be marketed in the UK, it must first be granted a marketing authorisation (MA) by the relevant licensing body, the Medicines and Healthcare products Regulatory Agency (MHRA). The term 'marketing authorisation' replaced the earlier term, 'product licence' (PL) in the early 1970s when the UK joined the European Economic Community (now the European Union) but PL still frequently appears on packs of medicines sold in the UK. Before granting an MA, the MHRA must be satisfied of the safety, quality and efficacy of the medicinal product. This is achieved by presentation of very large quantities of evidence derived from laboratory and clinical trials to demonstrate that the drug is both reasonably safe and actually achieves the medicinal purpose it claims to have and evidence of the manufacturing and quality control processes to ensure that the quality of the product will be consistent and reliable. Once the MHRA is satisfied (which can take many years from the development of the drug) the medicine is licensed.

## The importance of a medicine being licensed

We have drawn particular attention to the process of licensing because it affects the risks surrounding the prescribing of medicines. If a medicine is licensed, then provided the medicine is prescribed for the purposes, conditions and patients specified in the licence, the MA holder will be liable for any adverse effects that the medicine may have on the patient who takes it. The licence is, in effect, a guarantee from the MA holder direct to the patient that the MA holder will be liable for compensation for any unexpected harm (if proven) that arises when the medicine is prescribed and used according to the conditions of the MA. Note that this guarantee only applies when the medicine is prescribed and used 'within' the licence. You, as the prescriber, can rely on the MA holder for this protection.

It follows, therefore, that if you depart from the conditions specified in the marketing authorisation (variously called off-label, off-licence or outwith the licence), or prescribe something without a marketing authorisation at all (that is unlicensed), you as prescriber will carry liability for any harm that may result. For this reason it is very important that you are aware of the licensing status of any medicines that you prescribe. The important details of a MA or PL for most UK licensed medicines are set out in the Compendium of Data Sheets and Summaries of Product Characteristics (SPC) published by the organisation representing the pharmaceutical industry (ABPI or Association of the British Pharmaceutical Industry) (eMC, 2009). The SPC covers a great many matters: the presentation (tablet, capsule, liquid, cream, colour, shape, markings plus strength and dose volume); the indications or uses (which diseases in which patients); the recommended dosages and methods of administration; the contraindications (when not to use it) and warnings about side-effects as well as the legal category and the product licence number. If you prescribe any medicine in circumstances which are not clearly covered in this detailed specification, then the liability for safety of that medicine becomes yours. Such 'off-label' usage is actually quite common, say on paediatric wards, in palliative care or in dermatology.

In some circumstances (see later) non-medical prescribers can also prescribe unlicensed medicines – that is products or substances that have not been subject to any licensing process in the UK. This means that not only may their safety be suspect but also their quality and efficacy. One of the drawbacks of acquiring medicines over the Internet is the heightened danger of receiving medicines which are not in fact what they claim to be or worse, they may contain no active ingredient or harmful ingredients. If you are not a pharmacist, try the exercises in *Box 2.1* to help you understand the above points.

---

**Box 2.1** *Practical exercises on licensing and medicinal products for non-pharmacists*

1 Visit your local pharmacy and look at the medicines on open display. Look for the PL number or MA number and find out what the numbers represent.
2 Look at the shelves containing dental products and shampoos and find some with PL or MA numbers. Why do you think these products are licensed medicines?
3 Ask your pharmacy colleagues to show you a copy of the SPC compendium and look up the medicines that you are likely to be prescribing. Will they be fully licensed, 'off-label' or unlicensed?

You may find your pharmacist can help you to complete this exercise!

---

Before moving on to the supply of medicines you should be aware that the Medicines and Healthcare products Regulatory Agency (MHRA) is responsible for enforcing adverse drug reaction (ADR) reporting by MA and PL holders and for dealing with reports under the 'yellow card scheme' (samples are bound into the back of the *British National Formulary* – BNF). This is a system available to doctors, pharmacists, nurses and patients to report any ADRs associated with medicines, both prescribed and purchased over the counter and with complementary medicines and traditional remedies. Virtually all pharmaceutical companies belong to the Association of the British Pharmaceutical Industry (ABPI) which has a code of practice for the marketing of medicines. This is published in the SPC Compendium. You should recognise that, as a non-medical prescriber, you may be a target for promotional literature and visits by representatives of pharmaceutical companies.

## Legislation covering the supply of medicines

There are three categories of medicines under the Medicines Act:

- General Sales List medicines, GSL
- Pharmacy medicines, P
- Prescription Only Medicines, POM.

In addition, all controlled drugs are POM and CD. Each legal category of drug is subject to certain restrictions on their availability as follows.

### General Sales List (GSL) medicines

There are no restrictions on sale of these medicines except that they must be sold in the original manufacturer's packaging, there may be limits on the pack size and the sale has to be made from permanent premises, not from a market stall or van.

### Pharmacy (P) medicines

These can only be sold from a registered pharmacy under the supervision of registered pharmacists. Proposals have been made to change these restrictions but they should have little impact on non-medical prescribers. Part 3 Chapter 2 of the Health Act 2006 provides power to create a 'responsible pharmacist' for each community pharmacy and to amend the interpretation of supervision.

### Prescription Only Medicines (POM)

These can only be supplied or authorised for supply by an 'appropriate practitioner' (see below). A medicine is likely to be POM if:

- medical supervision is needed in use to prevent a direct or indirect danger to health
- it is widely and frequently misused
- it is a new active substance
- it is for parenteral administration (other than by mouth or the bowel).

Medicines are moved from one category to another. For example, the ulcer healing drug Zantac (ranitidine) started life as a POM, lower strengths were declassified as a P medicine and the lowest strength tablet is available as a GSL. The same drug may appear in all three categories but in differing strengths and pack sizes (e.g. ibuprofen). Changes in classification follow reappraisal of safety profiles and are effected through the marketing authorisation.

## Controlled drugs (CDs)

Mere possession of a controlled drug is a criminal offence unless you are covered by one of the exemptions in the legislation. The Misuse of Drugs Act classifies drugs into classes A, B and C; this has no relation to their use as medicines but relates to their relative harmfulness as illicit drugs, and is used to determine the scale of penalties for offences under the Act.

Controlled drugs are permitted to be used lawfully for medical purposes but are subject to further controls (in addition to those in the Medicines Act) depending on the category or Schedule in which they are listed. The five categories are described in *Box 2.2*.

---

**Box 2.2** *Controlled drug schedules*

- Schedule 1: Includes drugs with virtually no current therapeutic use, which are licensed solely for research purposes. An example would be cannabis or LSD. A Home Office licence is required for prescribing, possession and supply.

- Schedule 2: Includes opiates (e.g. diamorphine, morphine, pethidine and methadone) and major stimulants (e.g. amfetamine).

- Schedule 3: Drugs such as temazepam, buprenorphine and fluni-trazepam which are thought to be less likely to be abused than those in Schedule 2 and, if abused, are considered less harmful.

- Schedule 4: Contains two classes of drugs – benzodiazepines and anabolic steroids.

- Schedule 5: These are preparations containing CDs exempted from controls because of their low strength or concentration. Some are even exempted from POM controls and are P medicines. They have no special requirements as far as prescribers are concerned.

---

Only those drugs in Schedules 2 and 3 have relevance for non-medical prescribers. For the full details of controlled drug controls see Appelbe and Wingfield (2005) or the *Medicines, Ethics and Practice Guide* published annually by the Royal Pharmaceutical Society of Great Britain (RPSGB).

The legislation covering controlled drugs requires meticulous attention to detail and covers the following.

### Prescription writing requirements

We cover this later in the section on Writing prescriptions.

### Registers and safe custody

For Schedule 2 drugs, all transactions, both receipts and supplies, must be recorded in an official Controlled Drugs Register which may be computer produced as well as written and, although not yet a legal requirement, a running balance of the stock of each drug should be maintained. All Schedule 2 drugs (except secobarbital) and some Schedule 3 drugs must be kept in safe custody in a locked cabinet of a design approved by the police or, in the community pharmacy, in accordance with the specifications in the

Safe Custody regulations (Misuse of Drugs Act (Safe Custody) Regulations 1973 SI 1973 No. 798).

### Inspection and monitoring

Since 2007 (The Controlled Drugs (Supervision of Management and Use) Regulations 2006 SI 2006 No. 3148) all NHS and private health organisations must have appointed an 'accountable officer' who is responsible for the safe management of controlled drugs within that organisation. All healthcare providers who hold stocks of controlled drugs have to comply with standard operating procedures for their management and to make 'periodic' declarations that they have controlled drugs on their premises and the stock levels. Each primary care contractor (GPs, pharmacies, opticians and dentists) is subject to a formal controlled drug review once a year.

### Destruction

Stocks of controlled drugs that are unwanted, out of date or obsolete may only be destroyed in the presence of an 'authorised person'. The groups of people who are authorised to witness destruction of controlled drugs expanded in 2007 to include any officer of a healthcare organisation, including strategic health authority pharmacy leads, medical directors and clinical governance leads provided they are not themselves routinely involved in the management or use of controlled drugs.

### Appropriate practitioner

In the original Medicines Act Regulations there were only three types of appropriate practitioners:

- doctors
- dentists
- vets.

Since the advent of non-medical prescribing (see *Chapter 1*) four more categories have been added:

- community practitioner nurse (CPN) prescribers (formerly called district nurse or health visitor prescribers)
- nurse independent prescribers
- pharmacist independent prescribers
- supplementary prescribers (includes nurses, pharmacists, physiotherapists, podiatrists and radiographers).

The first six categories of practitioners are independent prescribers. Using their personal professional judgement they can prescribe for patients under their care any medicinal product that the law allows them to. Supplementary prescribers prescribe within a treatment plan – the clinical management plan (CMP) – in partnership with the doctor and the patient. (The form of the clinical management plan appears in Schedule 3B to the POM (Human Use) Amendment Order 2003 SI 2003 No. 696.) As we said at the outset, the Medicines Act and Misuse of Drugs Act apply both to NHS and private supplies of medicines. Thus doctors can and do write private prescriptions in all classes of medicines for patients who choose or are obliged to pay for their medicines privately, P and GSL medicines are available for sale in community pharmacies and GSL medicines are available from a wide range of shops, newsagents, petrol forecourts and the like. Moreover, doctors and dentists are allowed to supply all drugs, including controlled drugs, to their own patients directly. The law does not, however, allow them to sell medicines to the general public.

As we said above, only doctors, dentists and veterinarians were appropriate practitioners under the original Medicines Act. In 1992 (The Medicines Act: Prescription by Nurses etc. Act 1992) and again in 2001 (The Health and Social Care Act 2001), powers were secured in new primary legislation to facilitate and set conditions for the development of 'non-medical prescribers' in England. (Note that the implementation of non-medical prescribing is devolved to the home countries and the terminology and systems in Scotland, Wales and Northern Ireland may vary slightly from the account given here.) A community nurse practitioner must be a first level nurse or registered midwife, be annotated as a CPN in their professional register and is limited to the CPN formulary. Nurse and pharmacist independent prescribers must be similarly qualified and entered in their register and after a course of training may prescribe from the relevant formulary in the *British National Formulary* (BNF). A supplementary prescriber must be a first level nurse or pharmacist or a registered midwife or chiropodist, podiatrist, physiotherapist or radiographer and annotated as such in their respective professional registers. In addition, the law requires that where non-medical prescribers are treating NHS patients, they must be employed by an NHS body such as a Primary Care Trust (in England), an NHS Trust or a GP practice.

The above account describes the underpinning framework for the prescription of medicines in the UK. Before turning to the detail of those arrangements for non-medical prescribers, we should briefly consider the role of the NHS in medicines supply.

## NHS regulations

Supplies of medicines within the NHS must comply with the criminal statutory law in the Medicines Act and the Misuse of Drugs Act but the NHS can also impose restrictions (through administrative law supplemented by internal policies and guidelines) on the use of some medicines by professionals who are employed by or contract their services to the NHS. Breach of these NHS regulations can affect an individual's employment status within the service, and a breach of contract by an NHS contractor can lead to financial penalties and loss of contract. The most common form of exclusion is the 'black-list'; a list of drugs and other substances not to be prescribed under NHS Pharmaceutical Services. Writing a prescription for a black-listed product is a breach of the NHS contract terms of service for the prescribing doctor and means that a pharmacist who dispenses the item will not be reimbursed by the NHS. Black-listed drugs are marked in the BNF by a symbol representing the word 'NHS' with a line through it.

Exclusion is also achieved through the use of formularies. Dentists treating NHS patients may only prescribe from a limited number of drugs in the Dental Practitioners Formulary. In the same way, the restrictions upon prescribing to NHS patients by community practitioner nurses or nurse or pharmacist independent prescribers are set out in the relevant formulary in the BNF publications. It follows that those same prescribers may prescribe a slightly wider range of medicines for private patients but, in so doing, they will incur greater liabilities for their outcomes and will be well advised to have their own personal professional indemnity insurance (see *Chapter 3*).

The BNF also lists 'borderline substances' which the NHS will only pay for if they are prescribed in circumstances when the Advisory Committee on Borderline Substances has advised they may be regarded as drugs. Examples include specialised food supplements for malabsorption syndromes or enteral feeds. You should also note the use of the 'black triangle' against some BNF entries which denotes a preparation which is 'less suitable' for prescribing than others. The BNF advises 'Although such preparations may not be considered as drugs of first choice, their use may be justifiable in certain circumstances.' You may have to justify your decision to use black triangle preparations.

## Who can prescribe what in non-medical prescribing?

At this point we must stress that the legislation in this area is constantly changing, though not as rapidly as it did in the first few years of non-medical prescribing. Readers are strongly advised to download the latest version of guidance from the Department of Health website (www.dh.gov.uk) to supplement the information below. For example, at the time of writing, a decision had been announced to allow community nurse practititioners to prescribe nystatin for oral thrush in neonates – an 'off-label' indication. Also the outcome of consultations were awaited to extend the range of controlled drugs that could be prescribed by nurse and pharmacist independent prescribers and to enable optometrists to become independent prescribers.

### Community nurse practitioners (CNPs)

The formulary available to CNPs comprises a small range of medicines with a larger range of dressings and appliance. All medicinal products must be prescribed by their generic names but dressings and appliances can be prescribed by their trade names.

### Independent prescriber

The definition offered by the Department of Health is that 'independent prescribing is prescribing by a practitioner (e.g. doctor, dentist, nurse or pharmacist) responsible and accountable for the assessment of patients with undiagnosed or diagnosed conditions and for decisions about the clinical management required, including prescribing' (Department of Health, 2006). Provided you have successfully completed the appropriate training and you are working within your own competency (see Clinical negligence below), as a nurse or pharmacist independent prescriber you may prescribe almost any medicine that you believe to be appropriate for your patients. There are three limitations: you may not prescribe unlicensed or black-listed medicines and you may only prescribe controlled drugs in certain circumstances (see the relevant formulary in the current BNF).

### Supplementary prescriber

Supplementary prescribing differs from independent prescribing in that the treatment regimen is initiated or suggested by a clinician or other independent prescriber (but not a nurse or pharmacist) who is responsible for determining what is wrong with the patient. As a supplementary prescriber, you may only prescribe medication within a patient-specific CMP which may include authority to alter doses or to stop medicines that are no longer needed. You may prescribe off-label, unlicensed medicines or controlled drugs if they are specified in the CMP, but not black-listed medicines.

## Legislation on other ways of supplying medicines

Although this book is directed at non-medical prescribers, it is important that you are aware of the variety of ways in which medicines, particularly those which are POM, can be made available to patients other than by a prescription. In some circumstances these routes may be more appropriate to the patient's needs and a more efficient use of time and resource. Full details of the legislation are given in Appelbe and Wingfield (2005).

## Supply under patient group directions

Patient group directions (PGDs, formerly called group protocols) allow a wide range of health professionals (pharmacists and registered nurses, midwives, health visitors, ophthalmic opticians, chiropodists, orthoptists, physiotherapists, radiographers, paramedics or equivalent, dieticians, occupational therapists, orthotists, prosthetists, speech and language therapists) to authorise supply of POMs to specified groups of patients without the usual need for an individually prepared prescription. The most common example of this would be the supply and administration of flu vaccine. Here, all patients identified as needing this treatment are grouped together as a whole and are defined by their need for treatment not their medical condition. A practitioner working under a PGD can therefore only supply a flu vaccination to the category of patient defined in the direction. PGDs are written documents which must be signed by a member of the healthcare profession supplying the medicine and a doctor and pharmacist. The legislation clearly defines what must be included in a written direction.

When supplying medicines using directions healthcare professionals must supply exactly as per the written direction. PGDs may authorise supply of GSL, P, POM and CD medicines in certain circumstances but they must be followed to the letter; there is no clinical freedom to change the specifications. It would be a criminal offence if a POM other than that stipulated in the PGD is supplied or if a condition is treated that is not specified in the PGD.

## Supply under emergency supply provisions

Community pharmacists working in community pharmacies may, at their discretion, use two exemptions from the usual requirements to have a prescription before supplying POMs: emergency supply at the request of the patient or emergency supply at the request of the doctor.

## Supply against a signed order

Doctors and dentists may purchase POMs from community pharmacies for use in their practice. These could be medicines that a GP would carry in his or her bag for emergency use, or medicines that a GP would use in clinics in a primary care setting. Signed orders for POM medicines must be signed by doctor or dentist, as purchase of POMs in this manner constitutes a private supply. Nurse or pharmacist independent prescribers (or supplementary prescribers) are not able to purchase POMs via this route.

### Supply against 'written directions' to supply (in hospitals only, sometimes called standing orders or bed charts)

The legislation allows hospitals to supply a POM in the course of its business against a patient-specific written direction of a doctor. The written direction does not need to comply with the requirements specified for prescriptions (see below), but does need to relate to a specific patient. The intention is to permit the supply of medicines against a patient's bed card or notes. Most entries on a patient's bed card are directions to administer, but providing the wording is clear they can be used as an authority to supply, for example, take home medication.

## Legislation on prescription writing

To be legally valid, prescriptions must comply with regulations made under the Medicines Act. If an invalid prescription is dispensed, the dispensing pharmacy or pharmacist commits a criminal offence. The Misuse of Drugs Act adds further legal requirements for controlled drugs; both the writer and the dispenser of an invalid prescription for controlled drugs commit a criminal offence. The following list applies to information which must appear on valid NHS or private prescription for a POM.

- A signature (in ink) from the prescriber. This is the only part of the prescription that must be written personally by the prescriber, everything else can be written by someone else, computer-generated, etc. The law also permits the use of electronic signatures in preparation for an electronic prescription service.
- The (practice) address of the prescriber.
- The date the prescription was written. Prescriptions for POMs are valid for six months from the date of writing.
- Particulars indicating that the prescriber is an 'appropriate practitioner'. NHS forms will normally bear your pre-printed details; a private prescription should indicate the qualifications of the prescriber.
- The age of the patient if under 12 years.

These are the only legal requirements. Surprisingly, essential information such as the name of the drug, the strength, dose and quantity, and the name and address of the patient are not required by the Medicines Act! In addition, for prescriptions for Schedule 2 (except temazepam) and Schedule 3 controlled drugs, the prescription must comply with the following:

- The signature must be in the prescriber's own handwriting. Computer-generated or printed prescriptions are allowed but the signature must be handwritten. If a prescription is handwritten then this must be the handwriting of the prescriber (not, say, a receptionist).

- The total quantity to be supplied must be specified in words and figures. Prescribing quantities solely by dose and length of treatment is not valid.
- The form of the medicine (e.g. tablets) must be specified. This applies even when there is only one form of a medicine and/or the form is implied in the name (e.g. MST Continus, Sevredol, Morcap SR, MXL).
- The strength of the medicine, if there is more than one, must be specified.
- A dose must be specified. 'As directed' or 'when required', etc. are not acceptable as doses, but 'one as directed' or 'two when required', etc. are.
- The limit of validity of the prescription is 28 days from the date written on the prescription by the prescriber – or can be a specified later date if initialled by the prescriber.
- The quantity of controlled drug prescribed should not exceed 30 days' supply.
- Repeat prescriptions are not permitted.
- Private prescriptions for controlled drugs must be written on the official form.
- The private prescriber's identification number should appear on the prescription (not the professional registration number).

Although not in the legislation, you should be particularly aware of the need to keep prescriptions and prescription pads secure. They should be treated like cheques in a cheque-book. In the wrong hands, a blank prescription is worth several pounds; if already signed, it is worth much more – never pre-sign prescriptions. Keep the pads secure, locked out of sight in your car boot, etc. If a prescription pad is lost or stolen, report the loss immediately to whoever issues you prescription pads. Fraud surveillance and detection measures are now in place in the NHS and particular care may be needed to check whether patients are truly exempt from prescription charges. Avoid signing exemption declarations on behalf of patients if at all possible.

Records should always be made, ideally at the time of writing, of the prescriptions you write. The record should clearly indicate the date, name of prescriber, name of item prescribed, quantity or dose, frequency and duration of treatment, and, if appropriate, strength, dosing schedule and route of administration. Details of the consultation with the patient and your prescribing authority should also be included.

## Accountability and non-medical prescribers

We have seen above that there is a significant quantity of complex statutory criminal law to observe as a non-medical prescriber. However, the criminal law cannot ensure that you are competent in your prescribing practice; other mechanisms are needed. We have already described how, if you are employed in the NHS, your employer will expect you to work within your competence and within any internal directions, policies, formularies, standard operating procedures, etc. that your employer expects to be followed. If you do this, then your employer will have vicarious liability for any harm to patients that may result from your practice. This means that in the event of a successful civil law action for negligence (see below), your employer will meet any compensation payments to the patient. If, however, you depart (without good reason) from these requirements, or if you are carrying out work that your employer does not know about, then you may be personally liable for any compensation payments. Even if the consequences are not this serious, you may find that you will still be subject to internal disciplinary measures or may jeopardise your promotion or even your job. If you undertake prescribing in private practice then you should always check what professional insurance is available to you and consider taking out your own.

All non-medical prescribers will have their own professional regulatory (registration) body. Such bodies can also hold you accountable for the quality of your prescribing. They will also expect you to observe any ethical or good practice codes relevant to your profession. Any departure from these may be regarded as indicating that your fitness to practise should be investigated and all professional regulatory bodies have powers to convene professional tribunals with powers to order suspension, restricted practice or removal from the register. The standards that the regulatory body will apply will accord with the standard of proof in a civil action for negligence.

## Clinical negligence

We can merely outline the principles of clinical negligence here but for our purposes, the concept of professional negligence involves the establishment of three legal principles:

1 that the professional owed a duty of care to the patient
2 that there was a breach of that duty of care (either by an act or a failure to act)
3 that the breach of care caused harm to the patient.

If these three matters can be established, then the patient (or client or service user) may pursue a claim for compensation in respect of the harm suffered. From the perspective of a non-medical prescriber, you will always owe a duty of care to your patient when you prescribe medicines for them. So the first test will always be met.

To determine whether a breach of this duty has occurred means that a standard of care must be established. Then a judgement must be made as to whether or not you, as a non-medical prescriber met the standard or, put another way, whether or not you have acted properly. For many years the expected standard would be expressed as the 'Bolam test' derived from an important case in 1957 (Bolam v Friern Hospital Management committee [1957] 2 All ER118). This case established a principle that 'a doctor is not guilty of negligence if he has acted in accordance with a practice accepted as proper by a responsible body of medical men skilled in that particular art.' Replace 'medical' with terms relating to your professions, ignore the sexism and the dated language and, with a minor extension in the Bolitho case (the body of medical opinion must also rest on a logical basis Bolitho v City and Hackney Health Authority [1997] 4 All ER), this is still the test applied in relation to most cases of professional negligence involving health professionals. This does not mean that the 'experts would have done the same thing, but they would regard the defendant's actions as within the range of acceptable practice' (Montgomery, 2003).

Since 1957 the professions and politicians have produced ever more explicit and transparent expressions of what the acceptable standard of practice should be. These may be found firstly in Codes of Ethics or Practice and associated guidance and within NHS instruments such as National Service Frameworks (NSFs) or guidelines produced by the National Institute for Health and Clinical Excellence (NICE). Moreover a significant source of appropriate standards may now be found within specialisms, many of which have set up consultant positions, 'special interest groups' or designated 'health professionals with special interests' (these standards also underpin clinical governance accountabilities, see *Chapter 3*).

The final test for professional negligence is to prove 'causation'. That is, that the failure in performance led directly to harm for the patient. Often this can be the hardest aspect of a negligence case to prove. Patients may be suffering from several diseases or conditions, or taking several different medications that will also cause them harm. Again, the evidence from 'expert witnesses' may be crucial in establishing the likelihood causing harm and the extent to which the failure of the health professional may have caused it. Ultimately, if causation is proved, the remedy is compensation to the 'victim' via a tariff of injuries and penalties set from time to time by the courts.

## Ethical aspects of non-medical prescribing

The prescription of medication for a patient is an intervention, albeit a rather mundane and non-invasive one. It is therefore important that the patient has been fully involved in, and consents to, the intervention. Space does not permit a full account of the legal and ethical ramifications of consent, particularly issues of capacity and who may make decisions for children and vulnerable adults with, say, learning disabilities, mental disorder or dementia. Readers are referred to their own professional codes, ethical textbooks or the guidance on consent available on the Department of Health website.

There are good reasons for regarding consent as an essential part of successful healthcare. The securing of consent for any health intervention, whether or not it involves physical contact, is essentially the embodiment of respect for the patient's autonomy. If you were the patient, you too would want at least the option of knowing what is wrong with you, what treatments might be available, what the pros and cons of such treatments might be, etc. – in other words the opportunity to be in control of your own treatment as far as possible. We know that patients get well or manage their condition better if they fully understand, have agreed to and have confidence in their treatment. This happy position is called 'concordance' and is the ideal manifestation of properly obtained valid consent. In law, for consent to be valid, the person giving consent must:

- have capacity (be competent) to use and weigh up the information necessary to make the decision
- be under no duress, coercion or pressure to give consent (and may refuse)
- be provided with sufficient information in an understandable form to enable them to make the decision.

So, when taking the decision to prescribe medicines you will want to ensure that the information you provide is clear and accurate; you have covered the risks and benefits of the treatment; you have discussed possible alternatives including no treatment; you have allowed for poor sight, hearing or language difficulties in the patient; you have given time to absorb the information and deal with any questions from the patient and that you have checked the understanding of the patient by perhaps asking them to tell you what they believe they are consenting to.

A further ethical consideration is the need to maintain confidentiality of the information you handle or record as part of your prescribing process and to ensure privacy in your discussions with patients. Consent is not strictly necessary if you need to share information that is necessary for the patient's care with a fellow professional. However, you should aim to involve the patient by explaining who you may share their information with, exactly what information and why. Many aspects of confidentiality are now the subject of legal requirements, such as data protection legislation or statutes which require or permit disclosure without the patient's consent in certain circumstances. Again it is not possible to give a full account of these here but readers should refer to their own professional codes etc. as before. Of particular value is the NHS Code of Practice on Confidentiality available on the Department of Health website (www.dh.gov.uk).

## Conclusion

We hope the above account is not seen as a deterrent to non-medical prescribing! Only by knowing what the rules and risks are can you manage them and feel confident that you are a competent and safe prescriber. We help you to do this in the next chapter on the risk management and patient safety components of clinical governance.

## Further reading

### Websites

Department of Health. http://www.dh.gov.uk. The Department of Health site contains comprehensive information on the non-medical prescribing programme. It includes who can prescribe what, details of funding and training, information about prescriptions forms, good practice and ethics issues, liability, budget setting and monitoring.
Nursing and Midwifery Council. http://www.nmc-uk.org. The Nursing and Midwifery Council (formerly the UKCC) which maintains details of nurses and their prescribing authorities.
National Prescribing Centre. http://www.npc.co.uk/nurse_pres.htm. Contains vast quantities of prescribing support data and guidelines for assessing competencies of nurse prescribers.
Royal Pharmaceutical Society of Great Britain. www.rpsgb.org.

### Reference books

ABPI. *Medicines Compendium of Data Sheets and Summaries of Product Characteristics.* http://emc.medicines.org.uk.
Appelbe G E and Wingfield J (2009). *Dale and Appelbe's Pharmacy Law and Ethics.* London: Pharmaceutical Press.
Department of Health (2008). *Drug Tariff: National Health Service, England and Wales.* London: The Stationery Office.
eMC. *Patient Information Leaflet Compendium.* http://emc.medicines.org.uk/
Grice P (2007). *Chemist and Druggist Guide to OTC Medicines.* London: CMPMedica Ltd.
Joint Formulary Committee (2008). *British National Formulary (BNF)*, No. 56. London: British Medical Association and Royal Pharmaceutical Society of Great Britain.
*Monthly Index of Medical Specialities (MIMS).* London: Haymarket Medical Media.
Proprietary Association of Great Britain (2007/2008). *OTC Directory.* London: Proprietary Association of Great Britain (PAGB).
Royal Pharmaceutical Society of Great Britain (2002). *Medicines, Ethics, and Practice: A Guide for Pharmacists.* London: Royal Pharmaceutical Society of Great Britain.
Sweetman S C (2007). *Martindale: the Complete Drug Reference*, 35th edn. London: Pharmaceutical Press.
Wingfield J, Badcott D and Appelbe G E (2007). *Pharmacy Ethics and Decision Making.* London: Pharmaceutical Press.

## Periodicals

Carrying updates to medicinal products and their categories:
*Chemist and Druggist*
*Pharmaceutical Journal*

# References

Appelbe G E and Wingfield J (2005). *Dale and Appelbe's Pharmacy Law and Ethics*, 8th edn. London: Pharmaceutical Press.

eMC (2009). Compendium of data sheets and summaries of product characteristics. http://emc.medicines.org.uk/ (accessed February 2009).

Department of Health (2006). Improving patients' access to medicines: A guide to implementing nurse and pharmacist independent prescribing within the NHS in England. http://www. dh.gov.uk/en/Publicationsandstatistics/Publications/PublicationsPolicyAndGuidance/DH_4 133743 (accessed February 2009).

Montgomery J (2003) *Healthcare Law*, 2nd edn. Oxford: Oxford University Press, pp. 169–170.

# 3

# Clinical governance and patient safety in prescribing

*Richard O'Neill*

---

**Key learning points:**

- Define the concept of clinical governance

- Understand how the clinical governance framework supports prescribing in practice

- Describe the professional standards and competency that underpin non-medical prescribing by different health professionals.

---

## Introduction

Clinical governance is about ensuring that patients receive the highest quality of National Health Service (NHS) care possible and is achieved by systems and processes within the organisation for monitoring and improving services. The principles of clinical governance apply to all who provide or manage patient care services in the NHS. Quality is a fundamental goal in healthcare provision: it protects patients, individual clinicians, as well as the organisation. NHS hospitals and primary care services are required to create a culture together with systems and methods of working that ensure continuous quality improvement. Non-medical prescribing (NMP), patient group directions (PGDs) and minor ailment schemes (MAS) are all part of a range of NHS reforms designed to increase patients' choice and improve patients' access to medicines; utilise the skills of health professionals more effectively; develop more flexible team working; and ensure provision of more accessible and effective patient care. Successful implementation requires robust clinical governance mechanisms and effective team working to ensure high-quality care and patient safety.

## Clinical governance

Clinical governance is a comprehensive framework for improving the standard of clinical practice and healthcare. The Department of Health (1997) *The New NHS: Modern, Dependable*, established clinical governance in the NHS in 1997 as a national strategy to deal with failures in the quality of healthcare.

> *Clinical governance is a framework through which NHS organisations are accountable for continuously improving the quality of their services and safeguarding high standards of care by creating an environment in which excellence in clinical care will flourish. (Department of Health, 1998)*

With echoes of corporate governance (an initiative aimed at redressing failed standards in the business world), clinical governance was first addressed by the World Health Organization (WHO, 1985) in describing a multidimensional concept based on the provision of high-quality health. Four key dimensions of quality were identified: professional performance (technical quality), resource use (efficiency), risk management (the risk of injury or illness associated with the service provided) and patient satisfaction with the service provided.

A fundamental feature is the concept of an integrated approach to care. Clinical governance is designed to integrate, consolidate, codify and universalise fragmented policies and approaches to quality improvement (Scally and Donaldson, 1998). Activities, including clinical audit, continuing professional development, clinical guidelines/evidence-based practice, research and development, and effective monitoring of clinical care, became part of clinical governance.

Another fundamental requirement is the ability to implement change and make continuous improvement.

Clinical governance was initially underpinned by components known as the 'seven pillars of clinical governance':

1 Patient, user and carer involvement
2 Risk management
3 Clinical audit
4 Research and effectiveness
5 Staffing and staff management
6 Education, training and development
7 Use of information.

These components have been incorporated into the Department of Health's *Standards for Better Health* (Department of Health, 2004). The

Standards for Better Health (SfBH) form a key part of the performance assessment by the Healthcare Commission (HC) of all healthcare organisations and are divided into seven 'domains' designed to cover the full spectrum of healthcare as defined in the Health and Social Care (Community Health and Standards) Act 2003. Quality is embedded in the SfBH and they form the basis of an assessment framework that enables healthcare organisations to document evidence of good practice (Department of Health, 2004).

The seven domains are:

1  Safety
2  Clinical and cost effectiveness
3  Governance
4  Patient focus
5  Accessible and responsive care
6  Care environment and amenities
7  Public health.

Within the governance domain, healthcare organisations have to demonstrate managerial and clinical leadership and accountability, as well as the organisation's culture, systems and working practices, ensuring that probity, quality assurance, quality improvement and patient safety are central components of all activities of the healthcare organisation. This is achieved by applying the principles of sound clinical and corporate governance.

## Principles of clinical governance

The main components of clinical governance are:

- clear lines of responsibility and accountability for the overall quality of clinical care
- a comprehensive programme of quality improvement systems (including clinical audit, supporting and applying evidence-based practice, implementing clinical standards and guidelines, workforce planning and development)
- education and training plans
- clear policies aimed at managing risk
- integrated procedures for all professional groups to identify and remedy poor performance.

Non-medical prescribing, patient group directions and minor ailment schemes are well-established systems in the NHS for improving access to medicines. All of the components of clinical governance are relevant and must be present to ensure that non-medical prescribing enhances patient care without increasing risk or compromising safety.

## Clinical governance in community pharmacy

The Royal Pharmaceutical Society (RPSGB) policy paper *Achieving Excellence in Pharmacy through Clinical Governance* made recommendations to pharmacists, health authorities and others on clinical governance in pharmacy. It outlined the framework that was needed to be in place locally for clinical governance to be successful. It also identified where further development was needed and where pharmacists need support, such as: more effective integration of pharmacy into clinical governance structures; establishment of a programme of quality improvement activities (clinical audit, continuing professional development, implementation of clinical guidelines and evidence-based practice); and the development of policies aimed at managing risks and identifying and dealing with poor performance (Royal Pharmaceutical Society of Great Britain, 1999).

The Department of Health *Clinical Governance in Community Pharmacy: Guidelines on good practice for the NHS*, published in 2002 (Department of Health, 2002), established a plan to better integrate community pharmacy into the wider clinical governance agenda operating within the NHS. The guidelines addressed areas including: support and training to community pharmacies; improvement in the integration of community pharmacy into communication networks; and identification of priorities for future development.

Clinical governance is an essential requirement for the Pharmacy Contract in England and Wales (The National Health Service (Pharmaceutical Services) Regulations, 2005). Contractors will be expected to ensure that standard operating procedures are used, that adverse incidents are reported to the National Patient Safety Agency, that continuing professional development is undertaken by pharmacists, that services are audited (Pharmaceutical Services Negotiating Committee, 2004).

## Clinical governance in non-medical prescribing

Appropriately qualified nurses and pharmacists (and most recently optometrists) who have successfully completed a training programme accredited by their regulatory body (and are subsequently registered as such with that body) are able to prescribe independently. Nurse independent prescribers (formerly extended formulary nurse prescribers) are able to prescribe any licensed medicine (i.e. products with a UK marketing authorisation) for any medical condition within their area of competence, including some controlled drugs. Pharmacist independent prescribers can prescribe any licensed medicine for any medical condition within their area of competence, with the exception of controlled drugs.

Supplementary prescribers enter into a voluntary partnership with an independent prescriber (doctor or dentist), and with the patient's agreement,

| Table 3.1 Introduction of non-medical prescribers | | |
|---|---|---|
| 1998 | District nurse/health visitor formulary | IP |
| 2002 | Nurses: extended formulary | IP |
| 2003 | Nurses and pharmacists | SP |
| 2003–2005 | Nurses: extensions to formulary | IP |
| 2005 | Chiropodists/podiatrists, optometrists, physiotherapists and radiographers | SP |
| 2006 | Pharmacists | IP |
| 2006 | Nurses: full formulary including some CDs | IP |
| 2008 | Optometrists | IP |
| SP, supplementary prescriber; IP, independent prescriber. | | |

to implement an agreed patient-specific clinical management plan. *Table 3.1* provides a summary of the introduction of non-medical prescribers.

## Benefits of non-medical prescribing

Non-medical prescribing can:

- improve patient care without compromising patient's safety
- make it easier for patients to get the medicines they need
- increase patient choice in accessing medicines
- make better use of the skills of health professionals
- contribute to the introduction of more flexible team working across the NHS.

In order to fully develop safe, effective prescribing practice, practitioners need to achieve and maintain competency in this role. This necessitates an effective professional governance framework, appropriately designed training and access to robust, quality-assured support and continuing professional development materials.

## Principles of clinical governance and non-medical prescribing

### Education and training

Education and training are integral to all components of clinical governance. Professional bodies have developed curricula for the education and training of supplementary and independent prescribers and accredited prescriber training courses (see *Box 3.1*).

---

**Box 3.1** *The RPSGB Outline Curriculum*

The Royal Pharmaceutical Society of Great Britain (2006) Outline Curriculum for Training Programmes to Prepare Pharmacist Prescribers includes the following.

**Indicative content**

- Consultation, decision making, assessment and review
- Influences on and psychology of prescribing
- Prescribing in a team context
- Applied therapeutics
- Evidence-based practice and clinical governance
- Legal, policy, professional and ethical aspects
- Prescribing in the public health context.

**Evidence-based practice and clinical governance**

- Local and professional clinical governance policies and procedures
- Development and maintenance of professional knowledge and competence in relation to the condition(s) for which the pharmacist intends to prescribe
- The rationale for national and local guidelines, protocols, policies, decision support systems and formularies – understanding the implications of adherence to and deviation from such guidance
- Prescribing in the context of the local health economy
- Principles of evidence-based practice and critical appraisal skills
- Reflective practice and continuing professional development, support networks, role of self, other prescribers and organisation
- Auditing, monitoring and evaluating prescribing practice
- Risk assessment and risk management
- Audit and systems monitoring
- Analysis, reporting and learning from adverse events and near misses.

From Royal Pharmaceutical Society of Great Britain (2006).

---

## Continuing professional development

A key responsibility of all non-medical prescribers is to keep-up-to-date with clinical and professional developments; with best prescribing practice and management of the conditions for which they intend to prescribe. It is essential for professionals to reflect on practice and identify continuing professional development (CPD) needs – some of which will be relevant to their practice as a prescriber.

Continuing professional development is a responsibility of both individual and employer. Increasingly, health professions are mandating professional development for their practitioners. Commonly there is the requirement for a certain number of CPD hours over a specified period and the maintenance of CPD or personal development portfolio. Various sources of information include the National Institute for Health and Clinical Excellence (NICE), National Service Frameworks (NSFs), National Prescribing Centre (NPC), the National Electronic Library for Medicines (NELM), as well as those associated with the professional bodies such the Centre for Pharmacy Postgraduate Education.

## Competencies

The National Prescribing Centre (NPC), formed in April 1996 by the Department of Health, aims to promote and support high-quality, cost-effective prescribing and medicines management across the NHS, and help to improve patient care and service delivery. The Centre has produced documents outlining a framework of prescribing competencies which can be used, in both independent and supplementary prescribing (see *Box 3.2*). It also helps by providing therapeutic training to assist those with a prescribing role in maintaining their competence.

---

**Box 3.2** *NPC Competency Framework Documents*

- **January 2007:** A competency framework for shared decision making with patients: achieving concordance for taking medicines http://www.npc.co.uk/pdf/Concordant_Competency_Framework_ 2007.pdf
- **October 2006:** Maintaining competency in prescribing: An outline framework to help pharmacist prescribers – second edition (October 2006) (including a version for local adaptation) http://www.npc. co.uk/pdf/pharmacist_comp_framework_Oct06.pdf
- **July 2004:** Maintaining competency in prescribing – an outline framework to help allied health professional supplementary prescribers http://www.npc.co.uk/pdf/maintain_comp_in_presc_ ofthahpsp.pdf
- **May 2004:** Competency framework for prescribing optometrists http://www.npc.co.uk/publications/optometrist/optometrist.pdf
- **March 2003:** Maintaining competency in prescribing – an outline framework to help pharmacist supplementary prescribers http:// www.npc.co.uk/pdf/pharmacist_comp_framework_march03.pdf

- **March 2003:** Maintaining competency in prescribing – an outline framework to help nurse supplementary prescribers – update http://www.npc.co.uk/pdf/nurse_update_framework.pdf
- **November 2001:** Maintaining competency in prescribing – an outline framework to help nurse prescribers http://www.npc.co.uk/publications/CompNurse/maint_comp_in_prescrib.pdf
- **April 2000:** Competencies for pharmacists working in primary care http://www.npc.co.uk/publications/CompPharm/competencies.htm

**Other competency frameworks**

- **September 2005:** Monitoring and inspecting the management of controlled drugs – a competency framework (England) http://www.npc.co.uk/pdf/CD1_Competency_Framework.pdf
- **March 2004:** Patient Group Directions – a practical guide and framework of competencies for all professionals using patient group directions. http://www.npc.co.uk/publications/pgd/pgd.pdf.

The 2006 NPC framework for pharmacists aims to:

- Help ensure that pharmacist prescribers possess all the relevant competencies to undertake supplementary prescribing, and/or independent prescribing
- Inform the commissioning, development and provision of appropriate continuing education and training programmes for pharmacist prescribers
- Help pharmacist prescribers and their employers/managers identify ongoing training and development needs
- Support individual continuing professional development (CPD)
- Support professionals locally by providing a framework to help recruitment and selection procedures and to inform appraisal systems.

From National Prescribing Centre (2006).

The competency framework should be used in conjunction with the clinical governance framework developed by the relevant professional body, for example, the Royal Pharmaceutical Society's Clinical Governance Framework for Pharmacist Prescribers (Royal Pharmaceutical Society of Great Britain, 2007a) (see *Box 3.3*).

This identifies aspects of good prescribing practice found in other professional guidelines (General Medical Council, 2006). Key principles include keeping up to date and prescribing only in the patients' best interests. There is a need to maintain objectivity, and therefore prescribers should not treat

**Box 3.3** *Suggested indicators of good practice for pharmacist prescribers outlined in the RPSGB's framework*

The pharmacist prescriber:

1 Communicates with patients/carers in a way that allows the pharmacist prescriber to understand the patient's needs, concerns and expectations about their medicines and enables the patient to make an informed choice about their treatment (including the risks and benefits)

2 Prescribes within their own competence and within their own scope of practice

3 Prescribes safely, appropriately, clinically and cost effectively

4 Monitors responses to therapy and modifies treatment or refers appropriately

5 Does not prescribe for themselves or anyone else with whom they have a close personal relationship (e.g. family and friends), other than in an emergency

6 Develops an effective relationship with the wider primary care team

7 Writes prescriptions clearly and legibly, and ensures that they are identifiable as the prescriber. (Pharmacist prescribers should have their own prescription pad and preferably generate printed prescriptions)

8 Does not direct prescriptions they have written to their pharmacy or any other pharmacy in particular

9 Preferably prescribes only when they have access to an individual patient's main medical record at the time of prescribing. In the future this will be accessed via an individual patient's electronic patient record. This may only be possible once IT allows sharing of records

10 Makes a contemporaneous, comprehensive, clear record of their consultation and prescription for an individual patient in the main medical record. Where it is not possible for a pharmacist prescriber to make a contemporaneous record in the main medical record, they should make a contemporaneous record, which is then added to the main medical record within 48 hours of the consultation

11 Stores prescription pads safely and takes appropriate action if they are lost or stolen

12 Must not ask for or accept any inducement, gift or hospitality which may affect or be seen to affect their judgement when making a prescribing decision

13 Regularly participates in CPD relating to prescribing and maintains a record of their CPD activity within their CPD portfolio

14 Ensures separation of the prescribing and dispensing wherever possible. Where the pharmacist is both prescribing and dispensing for an individual patient, a suitably competent second person (as designated in the pharmacy Standard Operating Procedure) should be involved in accuracy checking of the dispensed medicine. If the pharmacist does both prescribe and dispense for the patient without the involvement of a suitably competent second person then records should be made to ensure good clinical governance and probity

15 Carries out any relevant physical examinations of patients competently and with regard to the patient's dignity and privacy.

### Additional indicators for pharmacist supplementary prescribers

In addition, the pharmacist supplementary prescriber:

16 Prescribes according to the clinical management plan (CMP) agreed with the independent prescriber, for an individual patient

17 Refers all individual patient circumstances that fall outside the clinical management plan, or outside the pharmacist supplementary prescriber's competency, to an independent prescriber who is responsible for that patient's care

18 Develops an effective relationship with the independent prescriber and participates as a member of the wider primary care team

From Royal Pharmaceutical Society of Great Britain (2007a).

themselves or someone with whom a close relationship exists. Prescribers also must not allow personal or employers' financial or commercial interests to influence prescribing. Prescribing situations that require special consideration include prescribing for patients to whom the prescriber also dispenses (as well as potential conflict or interests also recognising the increased risk of error when both prescribing and dispensing) or directing to any particular pharmacy; prescribing for special groups such as children; and prescribing unlicensed medicines (independent prescribers are not authorised to prescribe unlicensed medication) or medicines for use outside the terms of their licence (off-label). Prescribers must only act in the best interests of the patient and must be perceived to be doing so. Financial or commercial interest must not affect the way healthcare professionals prescribe. Prescribers must also be seen to be uninfluenced by any promotional activities or inducements associated with medicines and prescribing decisions. Pharmacists already prescribe, dispense and sell medicines, although not necessarily of uniform high quality or evidence based when it comes to over-the-counter (OTC) medicines (Watson and Bond, 2004), and are accustomed to dealing with any professional/commercial tension. Prescribers need to be able to recognise and deal with pressures from pharmaceutical companies, for example, or from patients that might lead to inappropriate prescribing.

Care must be taken to avoid any potential conflicts of interest associated with clinical judgements. This is emphasised in professional codes of practice (see *Box 3.4*)

---

**Box 3.4** *Professional standards and guidance for pharmacist prescribers (RPSGB)*

2.1.8 When prescribing unlicensed medicines or medicines outside their licensed indications ('off-label') you must be satisfied that it would better serve the patient's needs than a licensed alternative and ensure that the patient, or their representative, is aware that it is unlicensed or outside of licence. In the case of unlicensed medicines patient consent must be obtained.

2.6.4 You must make your choice of medicinal product for the patient based on clinical suitability and clinical and cost effectiveness. The decision must not be based on potentially biased information, fraud or commercial gain.

2.6.6 You must not prescribe for yourself.

2.6.7 You must not prescribe for anyone with whom you have a close personal or emotional relationship, except in exceptional circumstances such as:

- No other person with the legal right to prescribe is available and only then if that treatment is necessary to save a life, avoid serious deterioration in the patient's health, or alleviate otherwise uncontrollable pain.

From Royal Pharmaceutical Society of Great Britain (2007b).

---

### Professional standards for nurses

The Nursing and Midwifery Council Code of Practice specifies that all nurses must refuse any gifts, favours or hospitality that might be interpreted as an attempt to gain preferential treatment (Nursing and Midwifery Council, 2008).

In the *Standards of Proficiency for Nurse and Midwife Prescribers* (Nursing and Midwifery Council, 2006) similar points to those emphasised in the RPSGB standards are made (see *Box 3.5*).

---

**Box 3.5** *Standards of proficiency for nurse and midwife prescribers*

**Practice standard 11: Prescribing for family and others (excluding Controlled Drugs – see practice standard 16)**

11.1 You must not prescribe for yourself

11.2 You should never prescribe for anyone with whom you have a close personal or emotional relationship, other than in an exceptional circumstance

11.3 If a prescription is necessary you should refer this to be undertaken by another registered prescriber wherever possible

**Practice standard 17: Prescribing unlicensed medicines**

17.1 You must not prescribe an unlicensed medication as an independent prescriber

17.2 You may prescribe an unlicensed medication as a supplementary prescriber as part of a clinical management plan providing:

a) The doctor/dentist and, you acting as a supplementary prescriber, have agreed the plan with the patient/client in a voluntary relationship

b) You are satisfied an alternative, licensed medication would not meet the patient/client's needs

c) You are satisfied there is a sufficient evidence base and/or experience to demonstrate the medications safety and efficacy for that particular patient/client

d) The doctor/dentist is prepared to take the responsibility for prescribing the unlicensed medicine and has agreed the patient/client's clinical management plan to that effect

e) The patient/client agrees to a prescription in the knowledge that the drug is unlicensed and understands the implications of this

f) The medication chosen and the reason for choosing it is documented in the clinical management plan

**Practice standard 18: Prescribing medicines for use outside the terms of their licence (off-label)**

18.1 Off-label prescribing is where licensed medications are prescribed outside of their licence. There are a number of circumstances in which nurses may prescribe licensed medicines for the purposes for which they are not licensed (this is most likely to be the case when prescribing for children, see the Guidance below). It is possible under current legislation for nurse or midwife independent/supplementary prescribers to prescribe off-label as independent prescribers. However in order to do so you must ensure the following conditions are met:

a) You are satisfied that it would better serve the patient/client's needs than an appropriately licensed alternative

b) You are satisfied that there is a sufficient evidence base and/or experience of using the medicine to demonstrate its safety and efficacy. Where the manufacturer's information is of limited help, the necessary information must be sought from another source

c) You should explain to the patient/client, or parent/carer, in broad terms, the reasons why medicines are not licensed for their proposed use. See the Guidance below

d) You make a clear, accurate, and legible record of all medicines prescribed and the reasons for prescribing an 'off-label' medicine.

18.2 You may also, as a supplementary prescriber, prescribe a medicine for use outside the terms of its licence providing:

a) There is a clinical management plan in place, written in conjunction with the doctor/dentist and in voluntary partnership with the patient/client or parent/carer

b) A doctor/dentist takes responsibility for prescribing the medicine and you jointly oversee the patient/clients care, monitor and ensure any follow-up treatment is given as required.

**Practice standard 21: Gifts and benefits**

21.1 You must make your choice of medicinal product for the patient/client, based on clinical suitability and cost effectiveness

21.2 You must maintain a 'register of interests' within your own personal portfolio, which may be produced on request if required for audit purposes

21.3 You should adhere to local corporate policy when maintaining a 'register of interests'

From Nursing and Midwifery Council (2006).

## Quality improvement systems

### Clinical audit

Clinical audit is a cyclical process to monitor practice and to ensure that improvements to the quality of care are implemented; prescribers must reflect on their prescribing practice; this involves review of clinical performance, refining and measurement against agreed standards and may involve some form of peer review/clinical supervision.

The RPSGB have developed a number of audit templates which are available on their website: www.rpsgb.org/registrationandsupport/audit/.

Guidance to help pharmacists implement the clinical audit requirements of the new contract for NHS pharmaceutical services in England and Wales was published in the *Pharmaceutical Journal* in August 2005 (Practice and Quality Improvement Directorate, 2005).

An audit trail of prescribing actions must be maintained, for example, through the keeping of prescribing records in patients' notes. Also, audits could be expected to focus on adherence to prescribing protocols, the incidence, management and reporting of adverse events, and outcomes assessment.

The Clinical Governance Support Team (CGST) have developed a clinical audit handbook (NHS Clinical Governance Support Team, 2005).

### Evidence-based practice

Prescribers must keep up to date with local and national guidelines and standards must ensure that their knowledge, skills and performance are of a high quality, evidence based and relevant to their field of practice.

### Clinical standards and guidelines

Prescribers are increasing asked to justify their prescribing and are monitored for inappropriate or excessive prescribing. Those who do not follow national and local level guidelines, such as NICE guidance or NSFs, need to justify and document their reasons. Guidelines have typically changed from something designed to assist to becoming a standard. While their aim is to improve quality of care, there is always the need to consider the individual patient and the patient view may be important.

In January 2007, NPC Plus published a web-based competency framework entitled *A Competency Framework for Shared Decision-making with Patients: Achieving concordance about taking medicines* (National Prescribing Centre, 2007). This document presents a framework of competencies that can apply to any health professional engaging in discussions with patients about their medications to allow health professionals to develop their knowledge and skills to benefit patient care.

### Responsibility and accountability

In the broad sense, accountability is concerned with the overarching perform-ance management framework within an organisation that is coherent with the themes of clinical governance. Clinical governance emphasises the need for 'clear lines of responsibility and accountability for the overall quality of clin-ical care' (NHS Executive, 1999). A crucial element is also the authority conferred on the individual to act responsibly and accountably. All practi-tioners will recognise the new responsibilities that prescribing brings. Greater freedom to prescribe and supply medicines carries with it greater account-ability. Patient safety is paramount and it is vital that prescribers keep their skills up-to-date and are competent to make the prescribing decisions for the therapeutic areas within which they work. The system of professional regula-tion and, in the near future, revalidation, are linked to fitness to practice and are designed to ensure that patients can trust that the care they receive will meet certain minimum standards of safety and quality (Department of Health, 2006, 2007, 2008; Chief Medical Officer, 2006).

Healthcare professionals have a responsibility to a number of groups: patients, the public, colleagues, their profession, employers, as well as to themselves. Responsibility has both legal and moral perspectives. Legally, it is reflected in the law of negligence and morally in the trust that exists between healthcare recipient and healthcare provider. Accountability differs from responsibility in that it focuses on justifying and explaining actions.

The legal and professional responsibilities of healthcare professionals are principally to be found in four main areas: statute law, common law, professional regulation and professional guidelines. When standards fall below those defined in these areas, a professional can be accountable to:

- society → public law: 'criminal' law (e.g. gross negligence, manslaughter), statute law (e.g. Medicines Act; Data Protection Act) → criminal prosecution → conviction/penalty
- patient → common law → civil action (e.g. trespass to person; negligence) → damages
- profession/regulatory body → statute/subordinate legislation (e.g. Pharmacy and Technicians Order 2007, Nursing and Midwifery Order 2002) → professional misconduct/malpractice → disciplinary body hearing → removal from professional register
- employer → contract law → contract of employment → breach of fundamental term of contract with NHS Health Authority or Primary Care Trust (e.g. gross misconduct, incompetence) → disciplinary action → termination of employment.

These spheres of accountability are not mutually exclusive and a single error in prescribing if sufficiently serious could, for example, result in a practitioner being held to account in all four areas.

The law does not accept lack of ability, lack of knowledge or inexperience as a defence. The standard of care is that expected of a reasonably competent person occupying the post. However, the healthcare professional is judged on knowledge at the time he or she acted and can have a defence if a respected body of opinion would have acted in the same way. Not unexpectedly, the standard expected of pharmacists will be high. Pharmacists can be expected to understand more about the medicines, risks and benefits and their potential for interacting with other medicines, than many of the other new prescribers (Newdick, 2003).

The law is seen as providing minimum standards; professional and ethical dimensions look for the maximum. Thus, healthcare professionals are accountable for their acts and omissions and must work within their skills, knowledge and competence. It requires insight that comes from critical reflection for a healthcare professional to recognise when they are not competent to act. They have a duty of care to the patients and in such circumstances must refer the patient appropriately. Accountability cannot be transferred and healthcare professionals should not accept tasks they are not competent to undertake.

All prescribers require professional indemnity and must advise insurers of their prescribing practice. Prescribers have a duty to their employers to act competently and to use resources efficiently and effectively. Employers hold vicarious liability for the actions of employees provided they are appropriately trained and qualified and are prescribing within agreed guidelines as part of their professional duties and with their employer's consent.

Professional accountability is typically vested in the professional registering body and prescribers must act in accordance with their professions code of professional conduct. Prescribers, as with any member of a healthcare profession, are individually accountable to their professional body. The RPSGB's Professional Standards and Guidance for Pharmacist Prescribers (Royal Pharmaceutical Society of Great Britain, 2007b) and the Nursing and Midwifery Council Standards of Proficiency for nurse and midwife prescribers (Nursing and Midwifery Council, 2006), for example, expand on the principles outlined in the codes of ethics, develop the professional standards and explain responsibilities. See *Table 3.2* for the regulatory bodies for non-medical prescribers.

## Poor performance

The care, well-being and safety of patients is central to any healthcare professional practice. Legislative and regulatory measures alone are likely to

**Table 3.2** Regulatory bodies for non-medical prescribers

| Regulator | Healthcare professionals |
|---|---|
| General Medical Council (GMC) | Doctors |
| General Dental Council (CDC) | Dentists |
| Pharmaceutical Society of Great Britain (RPSGB), Pharmaceutical Society of Northern Ireland (PSNI) | Pharmacists[a] |
| Nursing and Midwifery Council (NMC) | Nurses; midwives; specialist community public health nurses |
| General Optical Council (GOC) | Optometrists; dispensing opticians |
| Health Professions Council (HPC) | Allied health professions – arts therapists; biomedical scientists; chiropodists/podiatrists; clinical scientists; dieticians; occupational therapists; operating department practitioners; orthoptists; paramedics; physiotherapists; prothetists/orthotists; radiographers; speech and language therapists |
| General Chiropractic Council (GCC) | Chiropractors |
| General Osteopathic Council (GOsC) | Osteopaths |

The Council for Healthcare Regulatory Excellence (http://www.chre.org.uk/) oversees and reviews the performance of the above.
[a] To become a General Pharmaceutical Council – GPhC.

be ineffective in maintaining professional competence and standards. Personal factors are essential in striving for professional and moral excellence. Professionals have a moral, if not legal, duty to take appropriate action to protect patients and the public when policies, systems, working conditions and the actions of others may compromise care or safety.

Competence includes not only core knowledge and skills and their integration into practice but also interpersonal skills, lifelong learning and professionalism. Monitoring of individual competence is an activity of regulatory bodies. The RPSGB guidance document *Identifying and Remedying Pharmacist Poor Performance in England and Wales* is intended to assist organisations to recognise poor performance and outlines the principles that employers, including the managed care sector (NHS), should apply in identifying and remedying poor performance (Royal Pharmaceutical Society of Great Britain, 2004). Continuing professional development (CPD) is a framework for the maintenance of professional competence of pharmacists.

In the case of doctors and dentists, the National Clinical Assessment Authority (NCAA) can give confidential advice and support to the NHS on how to manage those whose performance gives cause for concern. If a difficulty becomes apparent, the employer, contracting body or the practitioner can contact the National Clinical Assessment Service (NCAS) for help. The NCAS has launched a web-based toolkit to help NHS managers with the challenging job of managing performance concerns locally (www.ncas.npsa. nhs.uk/toolkit/introduction/) and guidance on understanding performance difficulties in relation to doctors and dentists (www.ncas.npsa.nhs.uk/ resources/directory-of-resources-to-support-doctors-and-dentists/).

## Risk management and patient safety

A knowledge and application of risk assessment tools must become part of a healthcare professional's skills. Risks can be considered as having a constant presence and risk management processes are needed to manage risk:

- step 1 – identify risk
- step 2 – analyse risk–potential to produce harm–likelihood and seriousness
- step 3 – manage risk–training; protocols; guidelines help eliminate/control risk–anticipate risk (e.g. equipment failure)
- step 4 – evaluation and reflection.

Pharmacy contractors under the NHS Contract are expected to be pro-active when it comes to consideration and prevention of potential risks (Pharmaceutical Services Negotiating Committee, 2004). They must demonstrate evidence of recording, reporting, monitoring, analysing and learning from patient safety incidents and are required to ensure that adverse incidents are reported to the National Patient Safety Agency (National Reporting and Learning System (NRLS) www.npsa.nhs.uk/nrls/reporting/). Pharmacists need to be competent in risk management, including the application of root cause analysis and to undertake significant event audit (Ashmore and Johnson, 2006).

Patient safety is the prime concern of everyone in the NHS. *An Organisation With A Memory* (Department of Health, 2000) recommended as one of its four key targets that there should be a 40% reduction in the number of serious errors involving prescribed drugs by 2005. *Building a Safer NHS for Patients: Improving medication safety* (Department of Health, 2001) outlined strategies aimed at reducing the occurrence of prescribing, dispensing and administration errors.

*Patient safety: the process by which an organisation makes patient care safer. This should involve: risk assessment; the identification and management of patient-related risks; the reporting and analysis of incidents; and the capacity to learn from and follow-up on incidents and implement solutions to minimise the risk of them recurring. (National Patient Safety Agency, 2004)*

The National Patient Safety Agency (NPSA) (www.npsa.nhs.uk) was established in 2001 to identify patient safety issues and find appropriate solutions. The NPSA was subsequently organised into three separate divisions, each with distinct functions:

- **Patient Safety Division** – this division has the aim of improving patient care through the analysis of patient safety incidents, rapid response to incidents and the development of actions, in partnership, that can be implemented locally, to build a stronger culture of patient safety.
- **National Clinical Assessment Service (NCAS)** – this division promotes patient safety by providing confidential advice and support to the NHS in situations where the performance of doctors and dentists is giving cause for concern.
- **National Research Ethics Service** – this division has the role of facilitating and promoting ethical research within the NHS while protecting the safety, dignity and well-being of research participants.

The NPSA *Seven Steps to Patient Safety for Primary Care* lists actions that organisations, staff and teams can take to improve patient safety (see *Box 3.6*).

---

**Box 3.6** *Seven steps to patient safety*

**Step 1 Build a safety culture** – Create a culture that is open and fair

**Step 2 Lead and support your staff** – Establish a clear strong focus on patient safety throughout your organisation

**Step 3 Integrate your risk management activity** – Develop systems and processes to manage your risks and identify and assess things that could go wrong

**Step 4 Promote reporting** – Ensure your staff can easily report incidents locally and nationally

**Step 5 Involve and communicate with patients and the public** – Develop ways to communicate openly with and listen to patients

**Step 6 Learn and share safety lessons** – Encourage staff to use root cause analysis to learn how and why incidents happen

**Step 7 Implement solution to prevent harm** – Embed lessons through changes to practice, processes or systems

From National Patient Safety Agency (2004).

---

Errors associated with prescribing can arise during any stages in the prescribing process; for example, the decision-making process, including defining the patient's problem (diagnosis), defining the therapeutic objectives, identifying treatment options and deciding on appropriate treatments; and the prescription-writing process. Errors frequently occur due to inexperience or when dealing with new practices or techniques (Weingart *et al.*, 2000).

*Human error is most likely with the inexperienced and overworked staff, in a stressful environment, struggle with unfamiliar problems, competing tasks, and incompatible goals. (Maxwell* et al.*, 2002)*

Rational drug use is concerned with the safe, effective, appropriate and cost-effective use of drugs. Safety can be considered from a number of perspectives, including the nature and severity of the disease, the availability of treatment options, and whether the aim is cure or the control of symptoms. All treatments have risks and involve a balance between the risk (harm) and the potential benefit.

*Prescribing is one of the most powerful tools that health professionals can use in tackling disease, and yet it is also an important cause of patient harm. To prescribe safely and effectively across all therapeutic groups requires high levels of knowledge and skill, and, even with many years of training, balancing benefits against risks can be difficult. (Avery and Pringle, 2005)*

Patient safety challenges include the need to access accurate information about both patient and drugs at the point of decision making as well as the need for communication with patients and other health professionals, monitoring of treatment and the checking for adverse effects. Concerns highlighted by the medical profession about the quality and safety of non-medical prescribing have included a lack of consultation/diagnostic skills and a lack of access to patient information (for example, see Avery and Pringle, 2005). Nevertheless, the comprehensiveness of the programme provided to non-medical prescribers may be contrasted with that provided for medical students (Ellis, 2002; Aronson *et al.*, 2006).

A further concern identified in an evaluation of extended formulary independent nurse prescribing in primary care undertaken by the University of Southampton was that only 5% of nurses had access to systems providing computer-generated prescriptions, thereby missing out on the potential benefits of computerised alerts for drug interactions and allergies (Latter *et al.*, 2005).

Timely and comprehensive information is essential to aid clinical governance. This should include:

- **information about patients:** medication and systems such as computers for prescribing including electronic patient medication records;
- **information about medicines:** electronic databases, including adverse incident reporting systems, to support informed/evidence-based clinical decision making;
- **information about guidelines, protocols and policies** to guide practice; and
- **information about systems and delivery of care** including staff competencies and skills; appraisal and personal development planning; patient complaints; and audit.

Prescribing errors can occur for a variety of reasons. These include inadequate knowledge of the patient and their clinical condition, inadequate knowledge of the drug, calculation errors, illegible handwriting, drug name confusion, and poor history taking. Personal and environmental factors such as fatigue and workload may also contribute to the likelihood of error. A prescribing error is potentially the most serious of all types of medication error as, unless detected, it might be repeated systematically over a prolonged period (Smith, 2004).

*It is important that all prescribers, whether doctors or, increasingly, nurses, pharmacists and other health professionals are aware of the principles of safe prescribing and of potential risks. (Smith, 2004)*

Errors in prescription writing may be due to poor communications, inaccurate transcription, or unsigned or illegible prescriptions. Errors on prescription are associated either with incorrect details (errors of commission) or with

**Table 3.3** Prescription errors

| Errors of commission | Errors of omission |
| --- | --- |
| Incorrect drug or indication for use | Absence of legal requirements |
| Incorrect drug/product name | Absence of dosage form or strength |
| Incorrect dosage form or strength | Absence of dose or dosage regimen |
| Incorrect dose or dosage regimen | Absence of quantity or duration of treatment |
| Incorrect quantity or duration of treatment | |
| Duplicate therapy | |
| Drug interactions | |
| Contraindications or inappropriate therapy | |

After O'Neill (2001).

incomplete details (errors of omission). The former present a greater threat to the safety of the patient if not identified and corrected and are less easy to identify (*Table 3.3*).

The separation between prescribing and dispensing is seen as an important component of the 'checks and balances' necessary to ensure that medication is safe and appropriate (Emmerton *et al.*, 2005).

The increased risk to patients from non-medical prescribers performing both processes has been highlighted in standards and guidance (see *Box 3.7*).

---

**Box 3.7** *Professional standards and guidance*

**Professional standards and guidance for pharmacist prescribers (RPSGB)**

2.6.2 You cannot both prescribe and dispense medicines except in exceptional circumstances e.g. where the need for the medicine is urgent and not to dispense would compromise patient care. You must have robust procedures in place to demonstrate the separation of prescribing and dispensing.

2.6.3 Where you are involved in both prescribing and dispensing a patient's medication, a second suitably competent person must be involved in checking the accuracy of the medicines provided, and wherever possible, carrying out a clinical check.

From Royal Pharmaceutical Society of Great Britain (2007b).

**Standards of proficiency for nurse and midwife prescribers (NMC)**

Practice standard 10: Prescribing and dispensing:

10.1 You must ensure separation of prescribing and dispensing when-ever possible, including within dispensing practices

10.2 In exceptional circumstance, where you are involved in both prescribing and dispensing a patient/client's medication, a second suitably competent person should be involved in checking the accuracy of the medication provided

From Nursing and Midwifery Council (2006).

---

Errors may be due to person or systems factors or a combination.

*Whereas followers of the person approach direct most of their management resources at trying to make individuals less fallible or wayward, adherents of the system approach strive for a comprehen-sive management programme aimed at several different targets: the*

*person, the team, the task, the workplace, and the institution as a whole. (Reason, 2000)*

The issue of duplicate therapy illustrates a systems type error. Patients may be consulting a number of different prescribers and each requires accurate and contemporary notes and a record of the medicines (prescribed and non-prescribed) they are using.

*As the number of prescribers increases, so does the risk of mixed messages, crossed wires and misunderstandings. Reasonable steps must be taken to recognise and deal with this risk. Systems must be introduced to monitor, manage and minimise the danger. (Newdick, 2003)*

Typically, many factors contribute to any prescribing error and it is only when the aetiology of an error is understood that appropriate corrective action can be taken to minimise the same risk happening again. Mechanisms do exist to record and consider the error and the steps taken to avoid it in future. Two key initiatives within the clinical governance framework have been the implementation of the NPSA's National Reporting and Learning system (NRLS) designed for anonymous reporting of patient safety errors and systems failures by health professionals across England and Wales and the provision of specialist training on root cause analysis.

## Conclusion

For healthcare professionals such as pharmacists, taking on responsibilities for prescribing and monitoring therapy can be seen as a natural extension to their existing role. Pharmacists already have expertise in drugs: doses, formulations, routes of administration, adverse effects, drug interactions and contraindications, pharmacokinetics and pharmacodynamics. Pharmacy education has become more patient-centred, evidence-based and with an emphasis on pharmaceutical care. Pharmacists are used to monitoring prescribing, making medication-related interventions and minimising risk; requiring insight into where errors can occur and a high risk aversion/safety focus. Similarly, nurses have had a key role in managing clinical risk, and ensuring safe and effective care. However, prescribing introduces new quality assurance issues. In being granted the right to prescribe, healthcare professionals must also accept the duties and responsibilities. Responsibility must be taken for the whole prescribing process, including diagnosis, prescribing and monitoring. Healthcare cannot ever be risk or error-free. Prescribing is a powerful tool in treating ill health and it is important that risks and errors associated with it are minimised at every point in the process by having a rigorous clinical governance framework in place.

# Further reading

National Treatment Agency for Substance Misuse (2007). Non-medical prescribing, patient group directions and minor ailment schemes in the treatment of drug misusers. http://www.nta.nhs.uk/publications/documents/nta_non_medical_prescribing_1207.pdf#.

## Department of Health (www.dh.gov.uk)

Department of Health (1997). *The New NHS: Modern, Dependable*. London: Department of Health.

Department of Health (1998). A first-class service: quality in the new NHS. Health Service Circular 1998/113. Department of Health, London.

NHS Executive (1999). Clinical governance: quality in the new NHS. Health Service Circular 1999/065. The Stationery Office, London.

Department of Health (2000). An organisation with a memory. http://www.dh.gov.uk/asset Root/04/06/50/86/04065086.pdf.

Department of Health (2005). Supplementary prescribing by nurses, pharmacists, chiropodists/podiatrists, physiotherapists and radiographers within the NHS in England: a guide for implementation. Updated May 2005. http://www.dh.gov.uk/PublicationsAnd Statistics/Publications/PublicationsPolicyAndGuidance/PublicationsPolicyAndGuidanceArticle/ fs/en?CONTENT_ID=4110032&chk=c4V6nR.

Department of Health (2006). Improving patient access to medicines: a guide to implementing nurse and pharmacist independent prescribing in the NHS in England. http://www.dh. gov.uk/en/Publicationsandstatistics/Publications/PublicationsPolicyAndGuidance/DH_413 3743.

Department of Health (2006). Medicines matter July 06 – A guide to mechanisms for the prescribing, supply and administration of medicines. http://www.dh.gov.uk/en/Publications andstatistics/Publications/PublicationsPolicyAndGuidance/DH_064325.

Department of Health (2006). *Extending Independent Nurse Prescribing within the NHS in England*. London: Department of Health.

Department of Health (2007) Clinical management plans (CMPs). http://www.dh.gov.uk/en/ Healthcare/Medicinespharmacyandindustry/Prescriptions/TheNon-MedicalPrescribing programme/Supplementaryprescribing/DH_4123030.

Department of Health. National service frameworks. http://www.dh.gov.uk/en/Healthcare/ NationalServiceFrameworks/index.htm.

Department of Health (2008). The non-medical prescribing programme. http://www.dh. gov.uk/en/Healthcare/Medicinespharmacyandindustry/Prescriptions/TheNon-Medical PrescribingProgramme/index.htm.

### *Department of Health websites on supplementary prescribing*

http://www.dh.gov.uk/en/Healthcare/Medicinespharmacyandindustry/Prescriptions/TheNon-MedicalPrescribingProgramme/Supplementaryprescribing/DH_4123025.

### *Department of Health websites on pharmacist independent prescribing*

http://www.dh.gov.uk/en/Healthcare/Medicinespharmacyandindustry/Prescriptions/TheNon-MedicalPrescribingProgramme/Independentpharmacistprescribing/index.htm.

### *Department of Health websites on nurse independent prescribing*

http://www.dh.gov.uk/en/Healthcare/Medicinespharmacyandindustry/Prescriptions/TheNon-MedicalPrescribingProgramme/Nurseprescribing/index.htm.

http://www.dh.gov.uk/en/Publicationsandstatistics/Publications/PublicationsPolicyAndGuidance/ DH_4006775.

http://www.dh.gov.uk/PolicyAndGuidance/MedicinesPharmacyAndIndustry/Prescriptions/Non
medicalPrescribing/fs/en.

## National Patient Safety Agency (www.npsa.nhs.uk/)

National Reporting and Learning System (NRLS). http://www.npsa.nhs.uk/patientsafety/
reporting/
National Clinical Assessment Service (NCAS). http://www.ncas.npsa.nhs.uk/.
NPSA Patient Safety Division. http://www.npsa.nhs.uk/patientsafety/.
National Patient Safety Agency. Incident investigation and root cause analysis toolkit.
http://www.npsa.nhs.uk/patientsafety/improvingpatientsafety/patient-safety-tools-and-
guidance/rootcauseanalysis/.
National Patient Safety Agency. Incident decision tree. http://www.npsa.nhs.uk/patient
safety/improvingpatientsafety/patient-safety-tools-and-guidance/incidentdecisiontree/.
National Patient Safety Agency. Seven steps to patient safety. http://www.npsa.nhs.uk/
patientsafety/improvingpatientsafety/patient-safety-tools-and-guidance/7steps/.

## National Prescribing Centre (www.npc.co.uk)

National Prescribing Centre non-medical prescribing site. http://www.npc.co.uk/non_medical.
htm.
National Prescribing Centre (2001). Maintaining competency in prescribing: an outline framework to help nurse prescribers. http://www.npc.co.uk/nurse_prescribing/pdfs/maint_comp_
in_prescrib.pdf.
National Prescribing Centre (2003). Maintaining competency in prescribing. An outline framework to help nurse supplementary prescribers: update. http://www.npc.co.uk/pdf/nurse_
update_framework.pdf.
National Prescribing Centre (2004). Patient group directions: a practical guide and framework
of competencies for all professionals using patient group directions Incorporating an
overview of existing mechanisms for the supply and prescribing of medicines.
http://www.npc.co.uk/publications/pgd/pgd.htm.
National Prescribing Centre (2004). Maintaining competency in prescribing: an outline framework to help allied health professional supplementary prescribers. http://www.npc.co.uk/
pdf/maintain_comp_in_presc_ofthahpsp.pdf.
National Prescribing Centre (2004). Glossary of prescribing terms. http://www.npc.co.uk/pdf/
glossary_prescribing_terms.pdf.
National Prescribing Centre (2004). Saving time, helping patients: a good practice guide to
quality repeat prescribing. http://www.npc.co.uk/repeat_prescribing/repeat_presc.htm.
National Prescribing Centre (2006). Maintaining competency in prescribing: an outline framework to help pharmacist prescribers, 2nd edn. http://www.npc.co.uk/pdf/pharmacist_
comp_framework_Oct06.pdf.
National Prescribing Centre (2007). A competency framework for shared decision-making
with patients: achieving concordance for taking medicines. http://www.npc.co.uk/
pdf/Concordant_Competency_Framework_2007.pdf.

## Royal Pharmaceutical Society of Great Britain (www.rpsgb.org.uk)

Interim Guidance from the RPSGB. Identifying and remedying pharmacist poor performance
in England and Wales. http://www.rpsgb.org.uk/pdfs/pharmpoorperf0501.pdf.
Royal Pharmaceutical Society of Great Britain. Clinical governance website. http://www.rpsgb.
org.uk/registrationandsupport/clinicalgovernance/.

Royal Pharmaceutical Society of Great Britain. Pharmacist prescribing. http://www.rpsgb.org/worldofpharmacy/currentdevelopmentsinpharmacy/pharmacistprescribing/index.html.

Royal Pharmaceutical Society of Great Britain. Audit resources. http://www.rpsgb.org.uk/registrationandsupport/audit/.

Royal Pharmaceutical Society of Great Britain. Continuing professional development. http://www.rpsgb.org.uk/registrationandsupport/continuingprofessionaldevelopment/.

Royal Pharmaceutical Society of Great Britain (2007). Fitness to practise and legal affairs directorate: Fact sheet seven. Patient group directions: a resource pack for pharmacists. London: RPSGB.

Royal Pharmaceutical Society of Great Britain (2007). Clinical governance framework for pharmacist prescribers and organisations commissioning or participating in pharmacist prescribing (GB wide). http://www.rpsgb.org/pdfs/clincgovframeworkpharm.pdf.

Royal Pharmaceutical Society of Great Britain (2007). Professional standards and guidance for pharmacist prescribers. http://www.rpsgb.org.uk/pdfs/coepsgpharmpresc.pdf.

### Nursing and Midwifery Council (www.nmc-uk.org)

Nursing and Midwifery Council (2006). Standards of proficiency for nurse and midwife prescribers. http://www.nmc-uk.org/aFrameDisplay.aspx?DocumentID=1645.

Nursing and Midwifery Council (2007). Standards for medicines management. http://www.nmc-uk.org/aArticle.aspx?ArticleID=2995.

Nursing and Midwifery Council (2008). The NMC Code of Professional Conduct: standards of conduct, performance and ethics for nurses and midwives. http://www.nmc-uk.org/aFrameDisplay.aspx?DocumentID=3954.

### Websites

Centre for Postgraduate Pharmacy Education. http://www.cppe.manchester.ac.uk/.

Clinical Management Plans Online. http://www.cmponline.info/.

College of Pharmacy Practice. http://www.collpharm.org.uk/.

Faculty of Prescribing and Medicines Management. http://fpmm.collpharm.co.uk/.

Department of Health e-guidelines. http://www.eguidelines.co.uk/.

General Medical Council (GMC). www.gmc-uk.org.

Healthcare Commission. http://www.healthcarecommission.org.uk/homepage.cfm.

Health Professions Council (HPC). http://www.hpc-uk.org/.

Medicines and Healthcare products Regulatory Agency. http://www.mhra.gov.uk.

National Electronic Library for Medicines (formerly Druginfozone). http://www.nelm.nhs.uk/en.

NHS Clinical Governance Support Team. http://www.cgsupport.nhs.uk/default.asp.

NHS Clinical Knowledge Summaries (formerly PRODIGY). http://cks.library.nhs.uk/home.

NHS Information Centre. http://www.ic.nhs.uk/.

NHS Knowledgeshare (evidence-based practice). www.knowledgeshare.nhs.uk.

NHS Litigation Authority. www.nhsla.com.

NHS Patient Group Directions. http://www.pgd.nhs.uk/.

National Institute for Health and Clinical Excellence (NICE). www.nice.org.uk.

National Library for Health. http://www.library.nhs.uk.

National Patient Safety Agency. http://www.npsa.nhs.uk/.

National Pharmacy Association. www.npa.org.uk.

Nurse Practitioner. http://www.nursepractitioner.org.uk/.

Nurse Prescribing. http://www.nurseprescribing.com/.

saferhealthcare. www.saferhealthcare.org.uk.

## Northern Ireland

Department of Health, Social Services and Public Safety http://www.dhsspsni.gov.uk/.
Non-Medical Prescribing. http://www.dhsspsni.gov.uk/non-medical-prescribing.

## Scotland

Scottish Executive. http://www.scotland.gov.uk/Home.
Scottish Executive Health Department HDL 2004 35: Implementation of supplementary
    prescribing for pharmacists. http://www.scotland.gov.uk/Publications/2004/06/19514/39164.
NHS Scotland National Education Scotland: Non-medical prescribing in Scotland. http://www.
    nes.scot.nhs.uk/pharmacy/prescribing/.
Scottish Intercollegiate Guidelines Network (SIGN). http://www.sign.ac.uk.
NHS Education for Scotland. http://www.nes.scot.nhs.uk/.

## Wales

Welsh Assembly. http://www.wales.gov.uk/index.htm.
Welsh Centre for Postgraduate Pharmacy Education. http://www.cf.ac.uk/phrmy/WCPPE/
    index.html.

# References

Aronson J K, Henderson G, Webb D J and Rawings M D (2006). A prescription for better
    prescribing. *BMJ* 333: 459–460.
Ashmore S and Johnson T (2006). Guide to significant event audit. *Pharm J* 277: 174–175.
Avery A J and Pringle M (2005). Extended prescribing by UK nurses and pharmacists. With
    more evidence and strict safeguards, it could benefit patients. *BMJ* 331: 1155–1156.
Chief Medical Officer (2006). Good doctors, Safer patients. http://www.dh.gov.uk/en/Publications
    andstatistics/Publications/PublicationsPolicyAndGuidance/DH_4137232.
Department of Health (1997). *The New NHS: Modern, Dependable*. London: Department of
    Health.
Department of Health (1998). A first-class service: quality in the new NHS. Health Service
    Circular 1998/113. Department of Health, London.
Department of Health (2000). An organisation with a memory. http://www.dh.gov.uk/asset
    Root/04/06/50/86/04065086.pdf.
Department of Health (2001). Building a safer NHS for patients: improving medication safety.
    http://www.dh.gov.uk/en/Publicationsandstatistics/Publications/PublicationsPolicyAnd
    Guidance/DH_4006525.
Department of Health (2002). Clinical governance in community pharmacy: guidelines on
    good practice for the NHS. http://www.dh.gov.uk/en/Publicationsandstatistics/Publications/
    PublicationsPolicyAndGuidance/DH_4008717.
Department of Health (2004). Standards for better health. http://www.dh.gov.uk/en/Publications
    andstatistics/Publications/PublicationsPolicyAndGuidance/DH_4086665.
Department of Health (2006). The regulation of non-medical healthcare professionals. http://
    www.dh.gov.uk/prod_consum_dh/groups/dh_digitalassets/@dh/@en/documents/digitalasset/
    dh_4137295.pdf.
Department of Health (2007). Trust, assurance and safety: the regulation of health professionals
    in the 21st century. Cm 7013. www.dh.gov.uk/en/Publicationsandstatistics/Publications/
    PublicationsPolicyAndGuidance/DH_065946.
Department of Health (2008). Pharmacy in England: building on strengths – delivering the
    future. http://www.dh.gov.uk/en/Publicationsandstatistics/Publications/PublicationsPolicy
    AndGuidance/DH_083815.

Ellis A (2002). Prescribing rights: are medical students properly prepared for them? *BMJ* 324: 1591.

Emmerton L, Marriott J, Bessell T, Nisen L and Dean L (2005). Pharmacists and prescribing rights: review of international developments. *J Pharm Pharm Sci* 8: 217–225.

General Medical Council (2006). Good practice in prescribing medicines. http://www. gmc-uk.org/guidance/current/library/prescriptions_faqs.asp#5j.

Latter S, Maben J, Myall M, Courtenay M, Young A and Dunn N (2005). An evaluation of extended formulary independent nurse prescribing. University of Southampton, Department of Health. http://www.dh.gov.uk/assetRoot/04/11/40/86/04114086.pdf.

Maxwell S, Walley T and Ferner R E (2002). Using drugs safely: undergraduates must be proficient in basic prescribing. *BMJ* 324: 930–931.

National Patient Safety Agency (NPSA) (2004). Seven steps to patient safety. http://www. npsa.nhs.uk/patientsafety/improvingpatientsafety/patient-safety-tools-and-guidance/7steps/.

National Prescribing Centre (2006). Maintaining competency in prescribing: an outline framework to help pharmacist prescribers, 2nd edn. http://www.npc.co.uk/pdf/pharmacist_comp_framework_Oct06.pdf.

National Prescribing Centre (2007). A competency framework for shared decision-making with patients: achieving concordance about taking medicines. http://www.npc.co.uk/pdf/Concordant_Competency_Framework_2007.pdf.

Newdick C (2003). Pharmacist prescribing – new rights, new responsibilities. *Pharm J* 270: 25.

NHS Clinical Governance Support Team (2005). *A Practical Handbook for Clinical Audit Guidance*. London: Clinical Governance Support Team.

NHS Executive (1999). *Clinical Governance: Quality in the new NHS Health Service*. Circular. HSC 1999/065. London: The Stationery Office.

Nursing and Midwifery Council (2006). Standards of proficiency for nurse and midwife prescribers. http://www.nmc-uk.org/aFrameDisplay.aspx?DocumentID=1645.

Nursing and Midwifery Council (2008). Gifts and gratuities. The Code: standards of conduct, performance and ethics for nurses and midwives. http://www.nmc-uk.org/aFrameDisplay. aspx?DocumentID=4176.

O'Neill R C (2001). Professional judgement and ethical dilemmas. In: Taylor KMG and Harding G (eds) *Pharmaceutical Practice*. London and New York: Taylor & Francis.

Pharmaceutical Services Negotiating Committee (PSNC) (2004). Essential service – Clinical governance requirements in the new community pharmacy contractual framework. http://www.psnc.org.uk/data/files/PharmacyContractandServices/EssentialServices/service2 0spec20es8202020clinica120governance20_v12010200ct2004_.pdf.

Practice and Quality Improvement Directorate RPSGB (2005). Guide to audit. *Pharm J* 275: 203–204.

Reason J (2000). Human error: models and management. *BMJ* 320: 768–770.

Royal Pharmaceutical Society of Great Britain (1999). Achieving excellence in pharmacy through clinical governance. Royal Pharmaceutical Society of Great Britain's policy on clinical governance. http://www.rpsgb.org.uk/pdfs/achieve.pdf; Achieving excellence in pharmacy through clinical governance. Royal Pharmaceutical Society in Scotland's policy on clinical governance. http://www.rpsgb.org.uk/pdfs/achiscot.pdf.

Royal Pharmaceutical Society of Great Britain (2004). Identifying and remedying pharmacist poor performance in England and Wales. Interim guidance from the RPSGB. http://www.rpsgb.org.uk/pdfs/pharmpoorperf0501.pdf.

Royal Pharmaceutical Society of Great Britain (2006). Outline curriculum for training programmes to prepare pharmacist prescribers. http://www.rpsgb.org/pdfs/indprescoutlcurric.pdf.

Royal Pharmaceutical Society of Great Britain (2007a). Clinical governance framework for pharmacist prescribers and organisations commissioning or participating in pharmacist prescribing (GB wide). http://www.rpsgb.org/pdfs/clincgovframeworkpharm.pdf.

Royal Pharmaceutical Society of Great Britain (2007b). Professional standards and guidance for pharmacist prescribers. http://www.rpsgb.org/pdfs/coepsgpharmpresc.pdf.

Scally G and Donaldson L J (1998). Clinical governance and the drive for quality improvement in the new NHS in England. *BMJ* 317: 61–65.

Smith J (2004). Building a safer NHS for patients: improving medication safety. http://www.dh.gov.uk/en/Publicationsandstatistics/Publications/PublicationsPolicyAnd Guidance/DH_4071443.

The National Health Service (Pharmaceutical Services) Regulations (2005). Part 4: Clinical governance, fitness to practise and complaints. Statutory Instrument 2005 No. 641. http://www.opsi.gov.uk/si/si2005/20050641.htm#sch1p4).

Watson M C and Bond C M (2004). The evidence-based supply of non-prescription medicines: barriers and beliefs. *Int J Pharm Pract* 12: 65–72.

Weingart S N, McL Wilson R, Gibberd R W and Harrison B (2000). Epidemiology of medical error. *BMJ* 320: 774–777.

World Health Organization (1985) The Principles of Quality Assurance – Report on Working Group Meeting Convened by Regional Office for Europe (Copenhagen) in Barcelona 1983. European Reports and Studies. Copenhagen: WHO (Available in *Qual Assur Health Care* 1989; 1: 79–95).

# 4

# Principles of prescribing and drug handling

*Soraya Dhillon, Andrzej J Kostrzewski and Kiren Gill*

**Key learning points:**

- Describe a rational approach to safe prescribing

- Explain basic pharmacokinetic principles in the context of prescribing

- Explain the role of adverse drug reactions and interactions in prescribing

- Apply basic kinetic principles to aid prescribing.

## Introduction

Health and disease management are key government priorities. It is clear that demand for health is increasing and health resources are prioritised to achieve maximum health gain. In the UK the government has substantially invested in health, almost doubling the expenditure in the past 10 years. Despite high levels of investment, demand for efficiency, productivity and the achievement of effective health outcomes for patients are continually under the spotlight. Healthcare reforms are focused on a number of key priorities:

- public health and disease prevention strategies
- patient safety
- service redesign
- emergency and elective redesign
- tackling health inequalities
- patients at the centre of health reforms.

Health professionals must ensure effective use of resources to achieve safe and effective health outcomes. Prescribing plays a key role in the achievement of health outcomes and effective use of resources (Department of Health, 2004). It has been extensively developed in the past 5 years, promoting supplementary and independent non-medical prescribing in order to improve access for patients and develop more effective chronic disease management.

Prescribing by non-medical practitioners must ensure that the practitioner has a thorough grounding in the underpinning biological science, chemistry and clinical pharmacology. Patient safety must be at the forefront of the prescriber's responsibility and extensive literature has been produced on prescribing problems. Clinically significant prescribing errors have been reported to occur in between 0.3 and 39.1% of prescriptions, many of which result in patient harm (Lesar *et al.*, 1997; Dean Franklin *et al.*, 2005).

Health professionals are concerned about this issue and it has been reported that currently 500 000–600 000 patients per year admitted to NHS hospitals in England and Wales may experience a patient safety incident. This may include untoward events and medication errors, some of these leading to morbidity and unexpected deaths of patients (National Patient Safety Agency, 2007). Although the true extent of medication errors is difficult to quantify, they are recognised as a concern. Estimates differ due to the variety of criteria and definitions used, but it has been reported that the incidence of medication error rates in hospitals ranges from 4.4 to 6.2 events per 100 admissions.

## A rational approach to safer prescribing

Coombes *et al.* (2005, 2007) have identified key training needs for non-medical prescribers which should cover the following:

- Prescribers must understand the medication management pathway and roles of medical, pharmacy, nursing staff and patients.
- Prescribers should understand the key risks and errors within the medication systems.
- Prescribers must ensure effective communication and assertiveness skills to escalate concerns with colleagues in the context of drug safety.
- Training must also encompass the principles of safe and effective prescribing, use of information sources and good oral and written communication skills for confirming and reconciling a drug history.
- Prescribers need to be able to identify drug-related problems, in particular to be aware of prescribing issues for high-risk drug groups, such as antibiotics (e.g. gentamicin), anticoagulants (e.g. warfarin and heparin), intravenous fluids and electrolytes, and variable dose insulin.
- Prescribers must develop key skills and knowledge to enable a systematic approach for safe prescribing, including communicating a decision to other health professionals and carers.

In summary, any prescribing decision must ensure that a patient receives the correct drug form, route, dose, frequency and duration, and that the right patient gets the right drug. Any prescribing decision should ensure fundamentally the rationale for a medication and that the patient understands and agrees with the prescribing decision.

Non-medical prescribers therefore need a key grounding in the principles of prescribing and understanding how to design and prescribe dosage regimens. The General Medical Council (GMC) in the UK recommends that graduate doctors have knowledge and understanding of 'the effective and safe use of medicines as the basis of prescribing' and the ability to write safe prescriptions (General Medical Council, 2002). The GMC has provided clear guidance to doctors on prescribing so that they provide clear explanation to their patients on prescribing decisions. The GMC has also established key standards of good practice (General Medical Council, 2006).

These principles form the basis for non-medical prescribing.

## Prescribing principles

The National Prescribing Centre (NPC) has developed a framework to support the principles of good prescribing for non-medical prescribers by providing signposts to aid their clinical decision making (National Prescribing Centre, 2008). The NPC identifies seven principles of good prescribing and provides sources of further help and information. The seven principles of good prescribing are as follows:

1 Examine the holistic needs of the patient. Is a prescription necessary?
2 Consider the appropriate strategy.
3 Consider the choice of product.
4 Negotiate a 'contract' and achieve concordance with the patient.
5 Review the patient on a regular basis.
6 Ensure record keeping is both accurate and up to date.
7 Reflect on your prescribing.

Pharmacists are trained in developing a patient-focused approach to prescription review and hence already use a number of the above principles as part of their routine clinical management. They also have a drug use process (six steps) which is a systematic review of a prescription and follows a stepwise process:

1 **Need for a medicine** – When faced with a clinical symptom pharmacists ask first whether this is a drug-induced problem from prescribed, over-the-counter or alternative therapies, including interactions, side-effects, adverse events from non-pharmacological treatments.

2 **Choice of a medicine** – If the assessment of the clinical symptom now requires management, the pharmacist considers choice of therapy using an evidence-based approach. How should this condition be managed and what is the evidence base for the choice of therapy? The prescriber must also consider polypharmacy by reviewing the patient's current medication to avoid inter-actions, safety netting for side-effects (e.g. if adding a diuretic is the patient already on similar medication and does it need to be potassium sparing?). Choice must also take into account co-morbidities. If one drug benefits a condition then this dictates the choice of therapy (e.g. in a hypertensive patient who also has prostate problems, choose an alpha blocker).

3 **Dosage regimen in terms of route, dose, frequency, duration** – Pharmacists use their knowledge of the product range in terms of formulation to advise on an appropriate route. The basis of this decision incorporates patient choice and how this fits the patient's lifestyle. The principles of pharmacokinetics are then applied to ensure that the patient is prescribed an optimal dosage regimen.

4 **Goals of therapy** – Pharmacists ensure they have identified the goals of therapy and have discussed this with the patient.

5 **Monitoring and review** – Pharmacist identifies what is monitored in terms of the drug and the patient. This identifies what is monitored, how often and how this links to review and management of the treatment to achieve effective goals of therapy.

6 **Patient education and counselling** – This covers lifestyle advice, medication counselling and ensuring the patient understands and is able to mange their medication appropriately.

The NPC also recommends the mnemonic 'WHAM' which is used by pharmacists in recommending over-the-counter (OTC) therapies and should be used to support prescribing decisions:

**W** – Who is it for and what are the symptoms?
**H** – How long have the symptoms been present?
**A** – Any action taken so far?
**M** – Any other medication?

Non-medical prescribers should thus develop their knowledge base in pharmacology and the sociology and psychology of medicine-taking behav-iours. Barber (1995) outlined the principles of good prescribing which strives to involve the patient in the process. Fundamentally, prescribing must ensure the four Rs:

- right drug
- right time
- right dose
- respecting the patient's beliefs.

## Design of dosage regimens for safe and effective prescribing

Pharmacokinetics is the fundamental science discipline that underpins applied therapeutics. Patients need to be prescribed appropriate medicines for a clinical condition. The medicine is chosen on the basis of an evidence-based approach to clinical practice and must be compatible with any other medicines or alternative therapies the patient may be taking.

The design of a dosage regimen is dependent on a basic understanding of the drug use process described earlier. When faced with a patient who shows specific clinical signs and symptoms, pharmicists must always ask: 'Is this patient suffering from a drug-related problem?' Once this issue is evaluated and a clinical diagnosis available the pharmacist can proceed to use the drug use process to ensure that the patient is prescribed an appropriate medication regimen and understands the therapy prescribed. In this way an agreed adherence plan can be achieved. Pharmacists using the drug use process should consider:

- need for a drug
- choice of a drug
- goals of therapy
- design of regimen
- route
- dose and frequency
- duration
- monitoring and review
- counselling.

Once a particular medicine is chosen, the principles of clinical pharmacokinetics should be applied to ensure that the appropriate formulation of drug is chosen for an appropriate route of administration. On the basis of the patient's drug-handling parameters, which require an understanding of absorption, distribution, metabolism and excretion, the dosage regimen for the medicine in a particular patient can be developed. The pharmacist will then need to ensure that the appropriate regimen is prescribed to achieve optimal efficacy and minimal toxicity, that appropriate monitoring is undertaken, and that the patient receives the appropriate information to ensure compliance. Clinical pharmacokinetics is hence a fundamental knowledge base that pharmacists require to ensure effective practice of pharmaceutical care.

## Adverse drug reactions and interactions

Prescribers need to consider that drugs may cause unwanted effects and hence need to consider both adverse drug reactions (ADRs) and, if a patient is on more than one medication, drug interactions (DIs). An ADR is a response that is noxious, unintended and occurs in doses normally used for treatment, prophylaxis or diagnosis of disease or the modification of physiological function (World Health Organization, 1975). This definition includes drug interactions but excludes overdose.

ADRs can be classified into two main types – types A and B. In addition adverse effects may occur due to chronic use and can be classified as type C – chronic (e.g. osteoporosis due to phenobarbital). Other adverse effects may not appear until after a period of time or even when the drug has been discontinued; these are termed type D – delayed reactions (e.g. impact of long-term steroids on fertility).

Type A ADRs are predicable and hence common. They are the result of the normal pharmacological profile of the drug resulting in an exaggerated therapeutic response. Type A reactions are usually dose related and a number have a pharmacokinetic basis. They show high morbidity and low mortality.

Type B ADRs are usually unrelated to the drug's known pharmacological responses. These reactions are bizarre and cannot be predicted (i.e. idiosyncratic). Type B reactions are usually unrelated to dose and often have an immunological basis. They show low morbidity but high mortality.

These effects can be classified according to their immunological basis:

- Type 1 immediate hypersensitivity (e.g. anaphylaxis results from the drug acting as a hapten or is antigen antibody reactions)
- Type 2 cytotoxic antibody (e.g. haematological reactions: antibody–antigen complex alters membrane-bound proteins and activates complement)
- Type 3 immune antibody–antigen complex deposition (e.g. serum sickness, immune complex and deposition, as in glomerular nephritis)
- Type 4 delayed-hypersensitivity activation of T lymphocytes (e.g. Steven–Johnson syndrome, a cell-mediated response).

Factors that may predispose patients to adverse drug effects include:

- age (ADRs are more common in the elderly and when prescribing in the young, especially neonates and young children)
- renal and liver disease

- heart failure
- nutritional status
- history of allergy
- multiple co-morbidity.

Prescribers need to take care when prescribing for patients at risk. For example, elderly patients may have altered renal function, may be prone to sensitivity reactions to neurological medications and are also more susceptible to falls from postural hypotension. Patients in intensive care and unstable will be more sensitive to the effects of medication. Any patient with impaired hepatic or renal disease will have altered drug handling. Patients with brittle disease need to have medication titrated and any change in drug handling can affect the management of these patients. Care is also required when patients have acute infections since this will affect metabolic capacity. Prescribing for neonates and children also requires careful dose titration.

## Drug interactions

Drug interactions occur when patients are on more than one drug and this alters the patient's response to medication. Drug interactions can be caused by pharmacodynamic or pharmacokinetic responses.

### Pharmacodynamic

Pharmacodynamic responses may be *direct* or *indirect*. Direct pharmacodynamic interactions can result from antagonism or synergism. For example:

- The effects of opiates can be reversed by naloxone.
- Flumazenil can be used to reverse the effects of midazolam.
- Steroids alter the rate of synthesis of clotting factors, and the interaction causes potentiation of the warfarin effect.

Indirect pharmacodynamic interactions can result in altered clinical responses to other drugs. For example:

- Diuretics are known to cause hypokalaemia. If this occurs then a patient may show increased sensitivity to cardiac drugs such as digoxin and antiarrhythmics despite normal drug levels. Hypokalaemia can also reduce the sensitivity to other cardiac drugs such as lidocaine and procainamide.
- Drug-induced ulceration (e.g. non-steroidal anti-inflammatory drugs (NSAIDs)) provides a site for bleeding in patients on anticoagulants.
- NSAIDs cause sodium and water retention and can antagonise the effects of cardiac drugs.

*Pharmacokinetic*

Pharmacokinetic interactions can be caused by alterations in the basic processes of absorption, distribution metabolism and excretion (ADME). See *Box 4.2* for a summary of basic clinical pharmacokinetics.

**Absorption**

Prescribers need to consider four basic mechanisms:

1 **Binding or chelation of drugs** – antacids, colestyramine, colestipol, bran and kaolin (e.g. colestyramine binds warfarin, nasogastric feeds bind phenytoin).

2 **Altered gastrointestinal motility** – metoclopramide, opiates and drugs with anticholinergic properties alter gut motility and hence can affect the transit time of other medications (e.g. metoclopramide and paracetamol to enhance the absorption of paracetamol).

3 **Altered gastric pH** – antacids and drugs that alter gastric pH (e.g. proton pump inhibitors). Antacids also affect enteric-coated preparations (e.g. causing degradation of the formulation).

4 **Changes at the gut wall** – metabolism in the gut wall (e.g. enzymes inhibited by monoamine oxidase inhibitors). High-dose antibiotics eradicate normal gut flora.

**Distribution**

Displacement from plasma proteins of one drug by another can cause clinical problems (see *Box 4.1*).

---

**Box 4.1** *Distribution example*

| Drug A | Drug B |
|---|---|
| 95% bound | 50% bound |
| 5% free | 50% free |
| | |
| Displacement | Displacement |
| 90% bound | 45% bound |
| 10% free | 55% free |
| 100% change in free fraction | 10% change in free fraction |

Drug A shows a 100% change in free fraction and drug B a 10% change in free fraction, however the displaced drugs (drug A and drug B) are then distributed and metabolised.

In this interaction both changes are 'transient' (distribution and elimination of free drug concentration), but if drug metabolism is inhibited then it is more likely that there is an increase in free drug concentration for drug A.

This only affects drugs that are strongly protein bound (97% or more), have a small volume of distribution and where drug metabolism is also affected in the interaction. Examples include chloral hydrate and warfarin, warfarin and sulphonamide, and phenytoin and sodium valproate.

## Metabolism

Prescribers need to be aware of any drugs that alter drug metabolism. If a drug causes enzyme induction then the metabolism of other drugs may be increased. This will result in lower therapeutic drug levels and hence a reduction in therapeutic response which could lead to therapeutic failure. If a drug causes enzyme inhibition then this will result in a reduction in drug metabolism of other drugs, which will increase the therapeutic drug levels and hence an increased or exaggerated response can occur, leading to toxicity. Common enzyme inducers and inhibitors are shown in *Table 4.1*.

## Excretion

Drug interactions in excretion can result from effects on either glomerular filtration, active tubular secretion or tubular reabsorption. Examples of drug excretion interactions include loop diuretics affecting lithium and gentamicin, resulting in lithium retention and toxicity and gentamicin nephrotoxicity; the effect of salicylates on methotrexate, resulting in retention of methotrexate and toxicity; the effects of quinine or verapamil on digoxin, resulting in digoxin toxicity.

**Table 4.1 Key drugs implicated in metabolism interactions**

| Enzyme inducers | Enzyme inhibitors |
|---|---|
| Rifampicin | Isoniazid |
| Phenobarbital | Chloramphenicol |
| Carbamazepine | Erythromycin |
| Phenytoin | Sodium valproate |
| Griseofulvin | Ciprofloxacin |
| Ethanol | Fluvoxamine |
| | Fluoxetine |
| | Ciclosporin |
| | Grapefruit juice |

A comprehensive review of ADR can be found in Lee (2006). Key reference resources on managing drug interactions are the BNF (Joint Formulary Committee, 2008) and Stockley (2007).

## Managing adverse drug reactions and interactions

1 Recognition – always remember to review the medications list, talk to the patient and review allergies
2 Ask for help
3 'ABC' – remember to review the patient, in severe cases always remember 'airway, breathing, resuscitation'
4 Stop the medication and treat
5 Remember to consult specialist services if required – poisons units or TOXBASE
6 Documentation
7 Inform the patient and educate to avoid it occurring in the future
8 Reflection and review of practice.

# Patient safety issues in prescribing

Prescribing errors have been extensively described in the literature. Human factors play an important role in managing and minimising errors.

Three major levels at which errors occur have been proposed by Reason (1990):

- the individual prescriber level
- the system level (i.e. within procedures and protocols)
- the organisational level.

### Individual prescriber level

An individual prescriber can make an error either from lack of knowledge and not recognising they need to check something or interpretation of inadequate information. Or they may lack of the appropriate skills to apply their knowledge when prescribing (Lesar et al., 1997; Dean et al., 2002). Recognising the level of competence is crucial in managing these decisions. It is clear that medical students and junior doctors lack the confidence, knowledge and ability to prescribe safely; studies have shown that these clinicians are under-prepared and supported in this role (Ellis, 2002). More importantly time and pressure, including multi-tasking and physical tiredness, all increase the risk of errors.

## System level

Medicines management is a complex system and the care pathway from a prescriber reaching a decision to starting therapy is complex. This pathway includes:

- decision to prescribe
- choice of regimen
- design of dosage
- dispensing and supply
- formulation and administration
- monitoring and review.

It is clear in this pathway of decisions that a number of health professionals are involved. From prescribing to the point a patient takes the medication has a number of steps, all of which have the potential for error and hence patient safety. Automation and electronic prescribing can influence a number of these stages and reduce the risk, and can lead to other types of systems errors.

## Organisational level

Various prescribing issues and problems have been identified over the past 20 years. Pharmacists record interventions and a number of studies have shown the benefits. There is, however, a medical culture in the prescribing process that focuses on drug selection. In most instances, senior clinicians advise on the drug choice and leave juniors to execute and complete the prescribing process. Checks need to be enhanced in the process, inculcating an opportunity for all to question the design of the regimen and choice of therapy. More emphasis is required on the administration, evaluation and monitoring of outcomes of prescribing decisions.

Organisations need to review their processes and support staff in prescribing decisions, especially junior doctors and new non-medical prescribers. There is also a need to review how prescriptions are written and managed and to look at discharge processes and transfer of information as patients move between and within healthcare sectors.

## Educational issues

It is clear that data are now emerging on the medicines that cause most problems in terms of prescribing (i.e. high-risk therapies that involve anticoagulants, insulin, fluids, electrolytes, antibiotics and analgesics). Prescribers must be up to date with alerts and always check routes of administration and drug dosing (National Patient Safety Agency, 2008).

Inculcating a patient safety culture and ensuring support for prescribers will minimise medication errors. Health professionals must ensure that they recognise their level of competence and always seek advice if they are not sure of a prescribing decision. Prescribing is an immense responsibility with multiple consequences. It is an extremely daunting experience which takes practice and experience to perfect. The key is to prescribe only when you feel confident to and are sure that what you are prescribing is correct. Check, check and check again! The points to remember are:

1 Know your patient – their medical history, their current medication and any allergies.
2 Know what you are prescribing and why – indication.
3 Decide on a drug of choice, route of administration, dosage – if unsure ask colleagues, ward pharmacist and consult your best friend the BNF!
4 Educate the patient – explain to the patient what has been prescribed and why.
5 Monitoring – if ward-based prescribing, inform nursing staff of changes, or if community-based inform the GP of changes.
6 If unsure of what to do, ask for help and be certain about your prescribing!

Helpful tips:

- Always have a BNF easily accessible.
- Ask colleagues if unsure – doctors, nursing staff, pharmacist.
- Practise and get a colleague to check – practice makes perfect.
- Know where protocols are kept – helpful aids.
- Keep a handy checklist of common things you prescribe.

## Conclusion

Non-medical prescribers need to ensure they have a thorough grounding and have confidence in understanding pharmacokinetics. Prescribers need to always apply the drug use process before making a prescribing decision and must always respect the patient's cultural and health beliefs. They must work within their level of competence and appreciate they have an ethical duty to keep patients safe, appreciating the factors that lead to medication errors.

## Case studies: Interpretation of drug levels as an aid to prescribing

The following case studies illustrate how an understanding of basic pharmacokinetic principles influence prescribing.

### Case study 1: Digoxin

An 84-year-old woman presents with increasing shortness of breath while walking around her flat. She lives alone, is independent and an ex-smoker. She is 81 kg in weight and 170 cm tall (67 inches). She comes to your pharmacy for a prescription of digoxin 62.6 µg daily.

Her past medical history reveals chronic renal failure, stage 4, stable creatinine 142 µmol/L; hypothyroid; atrial fibrillation; hypertensive; ischaemic heart disease; osteoporosis.

Current medication
- Aspirin 300 mg daily
- Adcal D3 2 tabs daily
- Imdur (isosorbide mononitrate modified release) 60 mg daily
- Levothyroxine 75 µg daily
- Omeprazole 10 mg daily
- Simvastatin 40 mg daily
- Senna 7.5 mg daily
- Furosemide 40 mg daily.

A week ago she was given a loading dose of digoxin and has been taking 62.5 µg daily for the last 14 days. After ringing her GP, you find that she has taken a digoxin blood level which is reported to be 1.0 µg/L.

**1 The GP asks whether he should increase the dose as the blood level is on the low side**

Her predicted glomerular filtration rate is calculated:

*Ideal body weight (IBW) = 45.5 kg + (2.3 × 7" > 5 ft) = 45.5 + (2.3 × 7) = 61.6 kg, compared to 81 kg.*

$$Creatinine\ clearance\ (Cl_{cr}) = \frac{[1.04\ (140 - 84)\ 61.6]}{142}$$

$$= 27\ mL/min$$

*Predicted digoxin clearance $(Cl_{dig}) = 0.053\ (Cl_{cr}) + 0.02\ (IBW)$ (on the assumption this woman has an element of heart failure)*

$$= (0.053 \times 27) + (0.02 \times 61.6) = 2.7\ L/h$$

$$C_{pssave} = \frac{(D \times S \times F)}{Cl \times \tau}$$

$$= \frac{(62.5 \times 1 \times 0.63)}{(2.7 \times 24)}$$

$$= 0.6\ \mu g/L$$

where $C_{pssave}$ is average steady state drug levels, $D$ is dose, $S$ is salt factor, $F$ is bioavailability, Cl is drug clearance and $\tau$ is dosing interval.

The predicted level is less than the measured level. This may be because:

- The level was taken less than 6 hours after the oral dose – This is possible and more difficult to confirm in primary care.
- Suspected non-compliance – This is also possible, as she is prescribed eight other medicines.
- Changing thyroid function – This is possible but unlikely from the patient's history.
- Congestive heart failure affecting renal function – This is also possible and the predicted renal function has deteriorated further.

A subgroup analysis of the Digitalis Investigation Group trial (DIG) suggested that participants over 65 years who had low blood levels (0.5–0.9 µg/L) had reductions in all-cause mortality (Ahmed, 2008). There has also been some suggestion that digoxin may be associated with an increased risk of problems in patients with atrial fibrillation (Gjesdal *et al.*, 2008).

Taking all these issues into account, the recommendation is to not increase the dose.

### 2 What other suggestions can you make regarding this woman's treatment?
You could suggest:

- adding ACE inhibitor with renal monitoring
- checking $K^+$ regularly
- reducing simvastatin dose to 10 mg daily
- repeating digoxin level in two weeks.

The patient should be counselled to recognise side-effects of digoxin toxicity, such as nausea, vomiting, constipation and disturbed colour vision.

### Case study 2: Theophylline

A 46-year-old man known to have brittle asthma. He is 183 cm tall and weight 84 kg. He is still smoking at least 20 cigarettes a day. He is not in distress and can hold a conversation comfortably. Peak flow is currently stable at 120 L/min. His past medical history reveals asthma since childhood. He has had numerous hospital admissions.

### Current medication
- Salbutamol nebs as required
- Symbicort 400/12 (budesonide 320 µg/formoterol 9 µg) 2 twice daily

- Theophylline 500 mg twice daily
- Tiotropium 18 µg once daily
- Prednisolone 40 mg reducing course
- Chewable vitamin D3 (Adcal D3) 2 daily
- Risedronate weekly
- EpiPen for emergency
- Montelukast 10 mg daily
- Metoclopramide 10 mg as required for theophylline sickness.

**1 What is the predicated level at average steady state?**
The predicted level at average steady state is as follows:

$$C_{pssave} = \frac{D \times S \times F}{Cl \times \tau}$$

Population Cl adjusted for a smoker:

$$Cl = 0.04 \times 84 \times 1.6 = 5.38 l/h$$

$$S = 1.0$$

$$F = 1.0$$

$$\tau = 24$$

$$C_{pssave} = \frac{1000}{5.38 \times 24} = 7.8 \ mg/L$$

**2 Level is reported as 4 mg/L what would you recommend?**
The reported level is 50% less than predicted. There are no drug interactions, according to the list given by the patient. The difference in the predicted and observed may be due to:

- reported level is incorrect
- patient adherence is suspect
- reduced bioavailability
- he is smoking more than he says
- combination of factors.

Recommendation:

- As the patient's peak expiratory flow rate (PEFR) is not deteriorating, maintain current therapy.
- Repeat the level.
- A cautious dose increment would be advised if the repeat level was confirmed. Increase night time dose to 750 mg and repeat trough at the morning dose to confirm.

## Case study 3: Phenytoin

A 31-year-old man known to have a cerebral glioma presents with seizures. He recovers from the acute episode and is discharged on the medications listed below. His past medical history reveals: nil. Allergy to penicillin.

### Current medication

- Phenytoin 400 mg daily
- Nicotine patches 14 mg/day
- Omeprazole 20 mg daily

Reported blood level of phenytoin is 4.8 mg/L (10–20 mg/L).

**1 Based on the reported level would you increase the dose? Explain your answer?**
The dose should not be increased at this stage. It is not known if this patient has been loaded with phenytoin and whether he is at steady state. Albumin status needs to be confirmed and the reported level adjusted if necessary.

The patient needs an urgent drug history and possibly a repeat level. Omeprazole may enhance the effects of phenytoin, although this mechanism is not understood. It is possible that if the dose of omeprazole is high enough, it may reduce the metabolism of phenytoin by CYP2C19. However, CYP2C19 has only a minor role in phenytoin metabolism (Stockley, 2007).

No interactions are listed with nicotine patches but animal studies suggest that nicotine may decrease the anticonvulsant effect of phenytoin (Czuczwar *et al.*, 2003).

## Case study 4: Phenytoin and theophylline

A 71-year-old woman presents with increasing shortness of breath while out shopping. She live alone, is independent and a smoker.

### Past medical history
- Left hemiparesis
- Hypertensive
- Smoker
- COPD
- No known allergies.

### Current medication
- Aspirin 75 mg daily
- Amlodipine 10 mg daily
- Phenytoin 300 mg daily
- Folic acid 5 mg daily
- Theophylline (Uniphyllin MR) 200 mg twice daily

- Symbicort 200/6 (budesonide 160 µg/formoterol 4.5 µg) 2 puffs twice daily
- Tiotropium 18 µg daily.

Blood level of phenytoin is measured as 5.1 mg/L. Blood level of theophylline is measured as 6.9 mg/L.

### 1 What is your interpretation of these levels?

It is unknown when these levels were taken in relation to the dose. You must have an albumin level in order to interpret this patient's phenytoin level. In this case it was reported as 31 g/L. Therefore the adjusted level is 7.1 mg/L.

- Reduced phenytoin serum levels: It has been found that higher serum levels of both drugs were achieved when the theophylline and phenytoin were given 2 hours apart.
- Reduced theophylline serum levels: Phenytoin is a known enzyme inducer, increasing the metabolism of theophylline by the cytochrome P450 isoenzyme CYP1A2. This can occur after about 5 days of therapy.

Other reports have shown that phenytoin can increase the clearance of theophylline up to 3.5 times. Theophylline dose may have to be increased by a factor of 1.5 to 2.

It has also been shown that the reduction in theophylline levels caused by phenytoin can be additive with the effects of smoking.

Note that theophylline itself can cause seizures, mostly in overdose, and should be used with caution in patients with epilepsy (Stockley, 2007).

### 2 The GP asks if he should increase the dose of both drugs as the blood level is on the low side

The answer is no. First check compliance. Blood levels of theophylline in COPD can be in the range of 5–20 mg/L.

It is suggested that the patient is counselled on taking the medicines at least 2 hours apart and the levels repeated in two weeks, pre-dosing.

---

### Box 4.2 Basic clinical pharmacokinetics

Clinical pharmacokinetics provides a basic understanding of the principles used to design a dosage regimen. Pharmacokinetics provides a mathematical basis to assess the time-course of drugs and their effects in the body. It enables the following processes to be quantified:

- absorption
- distribution

- metabolism
- excretion.

It is these pharmacokinetic processes, often referred to as ADME, that determine the drug concentration in the body following administration of a medicine. Non-medical prescribers need to have a basic understanding of these parameters in order to select and design an appropriate drug regimen for a patient. The prescriber needs to understand how some of these parameters can change (e.g. in the management of pharmacokinetic drug interactions or alterations in drug handling due to renal or liver impairment). The effectiveness of a dosage regimen is determined by the concentration of the drug in the body and usually this is measured in whole blood from which serum or plasma is generated. It is assumed that drug concentrations in these fluids are in equilibrium with the drug concentration at the receptor.

Measured drug concentrations in plasma or serum will be referred to as 'drug levels', which describes the total drug concentration (i.e. a combination of bound and free which are equilibrium with each other).

In routine clinical practice serum drug level monitoring and optimisation of a dosage regimen is only applied to drugs that show a narrow therapeutic range and for these drugs therapeutic drug level monitoring is required. For the majority of drugs, however, prescribers do not need to apply fundamental principals of pharmacokinetics since the drugs show a wide therapeutic range. *Figure 4.1* shows the serum concentration profile for a medicine that has a narrow therapeutic range, and impact of change dosage.

*Table 4.2* identifies the drugs that should be routinely monitored.

The principles described here, however, will provide an understanding of how drug-handling principles determine the design and development of a dosage regimen, and these principles therefore are applied to all drugs. The application of basic clinical pharmacokinetics in practice are described by Winter (2003) and Dhillon (2008).

### Basic principles

There are a variety of techniques available for representing the pharmacokinetics of a drug. The most usual is to view the body as consisting of compartments between which drug moves and from which elimination occurs. The transfer of drug between these compartments is represented by rate constants.

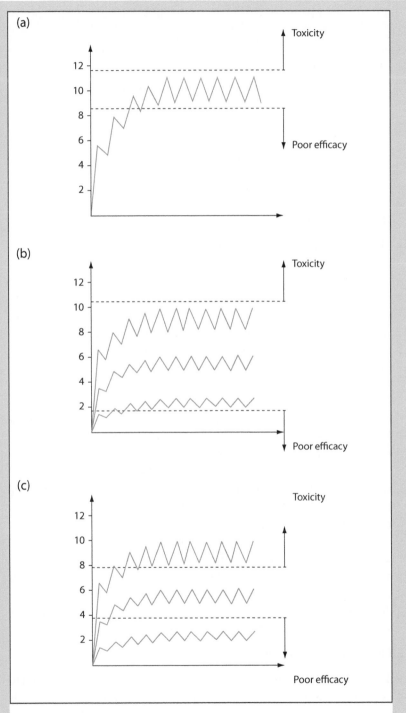

**Figure 4.1** Therapeutic range.

**Table 4.2** Therapeutic drug level monitoring – drugs that require assessment of plasma concentrations to optimise the dosage regimen

| Therapeutic group | Drugs |
| --- | --- |
| Aminoglycosides | Gentamicin, tobramycin, amikacin, vancomycin |
| Anticonvulsants | Phenytoin, carbamazepine, phenobarbital, ethosuximide |
| Cardioactives | Digoxin, lidocaine |
| Respiratory | Theophylline |
| Others | Lithium, ciclosporin, methotrexate |

## Rates of reaction

To describe the processes of ADME there is a need to consider the rate of these processes. Two basic concepts describe the rate of a reaction or process (any of the processes of ADME) which is defined as the velocity at which the reaction or process proceeds and can be described as either zero or first order. In a zero-order reaction the reaction proceeds at a constant rate and is independent of the concentration of drug A present in the body. An example is the elimination of alcohol. Drugs that show this type of elimination will show accumulation of plasma levels of the drug and hence non-linear pharmacokinetics. In a first-order reaction the reaction proceeds at a rate which is dependent on the concentration of drug A present in the body. It is assumed that the processes of ADME follow first-order reactions and most drugs are eliminated in this manner.

The majority of medicines used clinically at therapeutic dosages will show first-order rate processes (i.e. the rate of elimination of most drugs will be first order). However some drugs show non-linear rates of elimination (e.g. phenytoin, high-dose salicylates). First-order rate processes do not result in accumulation (i.e. as the amount of drug administered increases the body is able to eliminate the drug accordingly). Hence if you double the dose you will double the steady state plasma concentration. If the amount of drug is taken in overdose, however, then the elimination of the drugs will change from showing a first-order process to a zero-order process

### Elimination rate constant

This is the basic parameter for drug elimination ($k$) and can be used to estimate the amount of drug remaining or eliminated from the body per unit time. This parameter is also used to estimate the half-life of elimination.

## Volume of distribution

The volume of distribution $(V_d)$ has no direct physiological meaning, it is not a 'real' volume and is usually referred to as the apparent volume of distribution. It is defined as: that volume of plasma in which the total amount of drug in the body would be required to be dissolved in, to reflect the drug concentration attained in plasma.

The body is not a homogeneous unit, even though a one-compartment model can be used to describe the plasma concentration time profile of a number of drugs. It is important to realise that the concentration of the drug $(C_p)$ in plasma is not necessarily the same in the liver, kidneys or other tissues, etc.

$V_d$ is the constant of proportionality and is referred to as the volume of distribution, which thus relates the total amount of drug in the body at any time to the corresponding plasma concentration.

If the drug has a large $V_d$ that does not equate to a real volume (e.g. total plasma volume) it suggests that the drug is highly distributed in tissues. On the other hand if the $V_d$ is similar to total plasma volume it suggests that the total amount of drug is poorly distributed and is mainly in the plasma.

## Half-life

The time required to reduce the plasma concentration to one half its initial value is defined as the half-life $(t_{1/2})$.

This parameter is very useful to estimate how long it will take for levels to be reduced by half the original concentration. It can be used to estimate how long to stop a drug for if a patient has toxic drug levels, assuming the drug shows linear one-compartment pharmacokinetics.

## Clearance

Drug clearance (Cl) can be defined as the volume of plasma in the vascular compartment cleared of drug per unit time by the processes of metabolism and excretion. Clearance is constant for all drugs that are eliminated by first-order kinetics. Drug can be cleared by renal excretion or metabolism or both. With respect to the kidney and liver, etc., clearances are additive:

$$Cl_{total} = Cl_{renal} + Cl_{non\text{-}renal}$$

Mathematically, clearance is the product of the first-order elimination rate constant $(k)$ and the apparent volume of distribution $(V_d)$. Thus:

$$Cl_{total} = k \times V_d$$

Hence the clearance is the elimination rate constant (i.e. the fractional rate of drug loss from the volume of distribution).

Its relationship with half-life can be described by:

$$t_{1/2} = \frac{0.693 \times V_d}{Cl}$$

If a drug has a Cl of 2 L/h this tells you that 2 L of the $V_d$ is cleared of drug per hour. If the $C_p$ is 10 mg/L then 20 mg of drug is cleared per hour.

### Steady state

Prescribers need to determine the time to reach steady state and whether or not a loading dose is needed for a particular clinical situation. Most medicines are given as multiple doses hence providing the patients are given multiple doses before the preceding doses are eliminated accumulation of the medicine will occur until steady state is achieved. This occurs when the amount of drug administered (in a given time period) is equal to the amount of drug eliminated in that same period. At steady state the plasma concentration of the drug ($C_{pss}$) (i.e. fluctuations at any time during any dosing interval as well as the peak and trough) are the same. The time to reach steady state concentrations is dependent on the half-life of the drug under consideration.

### Bioavailability

Bioavailability ($F$) is the fraction of an oral dose which reaches the systemic circulation which following oral administration may be less than 100%. Thus, when $F = 0.5$ then 50% of the drug is absorbed. Parenteral dosage forms (intramuscular and intravenous) assume a bioavailability of 100%, and so $F = 1$ and is therefore not considered and is omitted from calculations. Prescribers in particular must be aware of changes in formulation for narrow therapeutic range drugs and when changing the route of administration.

### Salt factor

Salt factor ($S$) is the fraction of the administered dose which may be in the form of an ester or salt, which is the active drug. Aminophylline is the ethylenediamine salt of theophylline so that $S$ is 0.79. Thus 1 g aminophylline is equivalent to 790 mg theophylline.

### Population data

To apply the principles of pharmacokinetics in practice pharmacists can use population data. Population data are mean pharmacokinetic parameters that can be used to calculate predicted drug concentrations following a given dosage or to aim for a particular drug concentration and calculate a suitable dosage. Population data (i.e. basic pharmacokinetic parameters) can be found from standard reference sources or original pharmacokinetic studies.

## Further reading

Dhillon S (2008). Pharmacokinetics for everyday practice. http://www.thepharmacist.co.uk/clinical-services/pharmacokinetics-everyday-practice?page=0%2C0 (accessed 6 January 2009).

Evans W E, Schentag J J, Jusko W J and Harrison H (eds) (1992). *Applied Pharmacokinetics: Principles of Therapeutic Drug Monitoring*, 3rd edn. Vancouver: Applied Therapeutics Inc.

Winter M E (2003). *Basic Clinical Pharmacokinetics*, 4th edn. Philadelphia: Lippincott Williams and Wilkins.

## References

Ahmed A (2008). An update on the role of digoxin in older adults with chronic heart failure. *Geriatrics Aging* 11: 37–41.

Barber N (1995). What constitutes good prescribing? *BMJ* 310: 923–925.

Coombes I, Stowasser D, Reid C and Mitchell C (2005). Safely communicating the decision to treat through the implementation of a standard medication chart in all Queensland Health facilities [abstract]. Society of Hospital Pharmacists of Australia 27th Federal Conference, Brisbane.

Coombes I, Mitchell C and Stowasser D (2007). Safe medication practice tutorials: a practical approach to preparing prescribers. *The Clinical Teacher* 4: 128–134.

Czuczwar M, Kis J, Czuczwar P, Wielosz M and Turski W (2003). Nictoine diminishes anti-convulsant activity of antiepileptic drugs in mice. *Pol J Pharmacol* 55: 799–802.

Dean B, Schacter M and Vincent C (2002). Causes of prescribing errors in hospital inpatients: a prospective study. *Lancet* 359: 1373–1378.

Dean Franklin B, Vincent C, Schachter M and Barber N (2005). The incidence of prescribing errors in hospital in patients: an overview of the research methods. *Drug Safety* 28: 891–900.

Department of Health (2004). *Building a Safer NHS for Patients. Improving medication safety*. London: The Stationery Office.

Ellis A (2002). Prescribing rights: are medical students properly prepared for them? *BMJ* 324: 1591.

General Medical Council (2002). *Tomorrow's Doctors*. London: GMC.

General Medical Council (2006). Good practice in prescribing medicines. http://www.gmc-uk.org/guidance/current/library/prescriptions_faqs.asp (accessed 5 July 2008).

Gjesdal K, Feyzi J and Olsson S B (2008). Digitalis: a dangerous drug in atrial fibrillation? An analysis of the SPORTIF III and V data. *Heart* 94: 191–196.

Joint Formulary Committee (2008). *British National Formulary (BNF)*, No. 56. London: British Medical Association and Royal Pharmaceutical Society of Great Britain.

Lesar T S, Lomaestro B M and Pohl H (1997). Medication prescribing errors in a teaching hospital: a 9–year experience. *Arch Intern Med* 157: 1569–1576.

Lee A (ed.) (2006). *Adverse Drug Reactions*, 2nd edn. London: Pharmaceutical Press.

National Patient Safety Agency (2007). Medicines reconciliation. http://www.npsa.nhs.uk/corporate/news/guidance-to-improve-medicines-reconciliation/ (accessed 5 July 2008).

National Patient Safety Agency (2008). Prescribing issues. http://www.npsa.nhs.uk/search/?q=prescribing (accessed 5 July 2008).

National Prescribing Centre (2008). Non-medical prescribing. http://www.npc.co.uk/non_medical.htm (accessed 5 July 2008).

Reason J (1990). *Human Error*. Cambridge: Cambridge University Press.

Stockley I H (2007) *Stockley's Drug Interactions*, 7th edn. London: Pharmaceutical Press.

Winter M E (2003). *Basic Clinical Pharmacokinetics*, 4th edn. Philadelphia: Lippincott Williams and Wilkins.

World Health Organization (1975). *Requirements for Adverse Reaction Reporting*. Geneva: World Health Organization.

# 5

# Clinical decision making and evidence-based prescribing

*Maxine Offredy*

---

**Key learning points:**

- Understand the principles of clinical decision making

- Identify the component parts of the consultation

- Describe the importance of good history taking

- Understand the importance of non-medical prescribing

- Understand how errors and pitfalls in decision making can occur.

---

## Introduction

Clinical decision making, like prescribing, is a complex activity whereby healthcare practitioners determine the type of information they collect, recognise problems according to the cues identified during information collection, and decide upon appropriate interventions to address those problems (Tanner *et al.*, 1987; Offredy, 2002). Increasingly, these activities are required to be evidence based. Evidence-based medicine, which includes prescribing, has been defined as 'the conscientious, explicit and judicious use of current best evidence in making decisions about the care of individual patients' (Sackett *et al.*, 1996: 71). This implies that the notion of evidence-based decision making involves a combination formally acquired knowledge, experience gained from daily practice with patients and valid external evidence from research. It is the combination of these factors that identifies decision making as evidence based.

Clinical decision making involves different disciplines such as medicine, nursing, psychology, mathematical probability theory and economics. It should be noted that there is no one single accepted theoretical or research-based model of clinical decision making. The information used as currency in diagnostic decision making depends on clinical signs and symptoms and the results of investigation. Correct diagnosis depends on the accurate reporting of symptoms and recording of signs and the accuracy of diagnostic tests (sensitivity and specificity). In contrast, correct treatment decision making depends on due weight being given to the evidence available about the effectiveness, benefits and harms of different treatment. Evidence-based prescribing decisions therefore require a combination of clinical experience and sound knowledge based on the principles of clinical pharmacology (Maxwell *et al.*, 2002; Maxwell and Walley, 2003).

## Principles of clinical decision making

It is worth noting that the concept 'decision making' is not always clearly defined in the literature and is sometimes used interchangeably with other terms such as: clinical judgement, diagnostic strategies, clinical reasoning, diagnostic reasoning, clinical inference, reasoning strategies, clinical decision and human problem solving. Thus, an important aspect of the discussion on decision making is to define the meaning of the concept (Offredy *et al.*, 2008). For the purpose of this discussion, clinical decision making will be taken to mean the processes and procedures that healthcare professionals apply in order to reach a decision regarding the intervention to be used for the management or care of patients who consult them.

The literature on decision making can be divided into three major approaches:

1 **Decision analysis theory** (Raiffa, 1970) – also referred to as normative or prescriptive theory – involves statistical modelling of the decision-making processes; this may include Bayesian analysis. Decision analysis theory specifies how decisions *should* be made using various mechanisms such as decision trees and clinical policies (that is, protocols, guidelines and algorithms) as an alternative to the clinical or intuitive approach of how decisions *are* made. Decision analysis is a systematic approach to decision making under conditions of uncertainty (Raiffa, 1970). The uncertainty results from a variety of sources, some of which are outlined in *Table 5.1*. The key principle of decision analysis is that it is a method that aims to maximise the quality of individual decisions (including the patient's), thus promoting choice by providing different options. However, individuals can only select choices if they have been made available in the first instance and if the individuals are able to understand the data.

2 **Behavioural decision theory** includes social judgement analysis (Kahneman *et al.*, 1982; Doherty and Kurz, 1996); this is the observation of real-life decision-making processes, using predominantly experimental methods. The

| **Table 5.1** Sources contributing to uncertainty in decision making |
| --- |
| Errors in clinical data |
| Ambiguity of clinical data |
| Variations in the interpretation of data |
| Information overload |
| Differences in patient's and doctor's expectations |
| Uncertainty about the association between clinical information available and the presence of disease |
| Operational failures of, for example, testing equipment |
| Unreliable (and irrelevant) laboratory tests |
| Uncertainty about the effects of treatment |
| Uncertainty about relations between clinical information and the presence of disease |
| From Weinstein and Fineberg (1980), Schwartz and Griffin (1986). |

behavioural decision approach to decision making has its roots in Brunswik's (1952) probabilistic functionalism where he showed the importance of studying both cognition and context. Hammond's (1978) extension of Brunswik's work explored the traditional divide between intuitive and analytical thinking and rejected the view that these are dichotomous modes of thought (see Hamm, 1988, for a fuller discussion).

3 **Information processing theory** (Newell and Simon, 1972) uses process-tracing approaches combined with verbal data reports ('Think Aloud') (Ericsson and Simon, 1993) to explain human cognition (Offredy *et al.*, 2008). Newell and Simon's (1972) explanation of human thinking and problem solving proposed that these activities can be understood within the framework of information processing theory. The key principle of this theory is that it purports to provide an account of how people actually think and reach decisions, not how they ought to undertake these activities.

The first of these major approaches, decision analysis theory, provides a prescriptive view to decision making, while the last two, behavioural decision and information processing theories, are sometimes referred to as descriptive approaches to decision making.

Irrespective of the approach used, there are four key principles to decision making:

1 **Framing the problem**: this means developing a clear question from the problem identified, the purpose of which is to assist the decision maker

focus on the important aspects of the problem. This will mean that other issues of the problem will become secondary to the main point.

2 **Gathering information:** this refers to information that we know about as well as identifying or making estimates about what we do not know about the problem. Russo and Schoemaker (1991: 3) say that 'Good decision-makers manage intelligence-gathering with deliberate effort to avoid such failings as overconfidence in what they currently believe and the tendency to seek information that confirms their biases.' In other words, the decision maker should seek information to refute their views.

3 **Drawing conclusions:** the development of a clear question and good data or information does not equate to sound conclusions. A systematic approach to examining the literature is more likely to lead to better decisions than haphazard intuitive thinking.

4 **Learning from feedback:** this means that decision makers should establish a system to enable them to keep a record of the outcomes of their decisions and be willing to make adjustments accordingly (after Russo and Schoemaker, 1991).

These principles are embedded in the consultation and history-taking procedures, which form the topic of the next subsection.

## Consultation skills and history taking

The medical consultation is best described as a two-way interaction involving three components: the patient, the healthcare professional and the problem or illness under discussion. It is a set of skills that enables a person to convey information so that it is received and understood. History taking is an essential skill for health professionals in the management and treatment of their patients. The main aim of history taking is to assist in establishing a differential diagnosis. As with the patient consultation, history taking provides the opportunity for healthcare professionals to develop a rapport with the patient and contextualise the patient's problem within their life. History taking will also clarify the nature of the underlying pathological processes. It will inform about the illness as well as the disease. The illness (patient focus) is the subjective component and describes the patient's experience of the disease (the biomedical focus) (Shah, 2005). A key aspect in reaching an accurate diagnosis lies in obtaining a detailed description of the patient's symptoms during the consultation.

Historically, consultation processes have been researched from the perspective of general practitioners (GPs). However, since the 1950s many different models of consultation have been introduced due to the recognition of Balint's (1957) work in promoting a more patient-centred approach during the encounter with patients. He observed that the doctor's fixed style of consultation resulted from a combination of medical training, the doctor's beliefs about how sick patients should behave, how they should behave with doctors and how they should cooperate with their treatment. Balint was the first to recognise that the reasons given by the patient might not be the real ones for their visit and that the emotions triggered in the doctor could have an effect on the course of the consultation. Some of the models, based on the doctor–patient relationship primarily in GP practices, include the following:

- Byrne and Long (1976) identified six phases which form a logical structure to the consultation process. These were developed following analysis of over 2000 tape-recorded consultations and was the first to use the terms 'doctor-centred' and 'patient-centred consultation'.
- Pendelton *et al.* (1984, 2003) provide an approach to learning and teaching which describes seven tasks that form a comprehensive approach to the consultation. The model stresses the importance of the patient's view and understanding of the problem. The model also introduces the term 'consultation mapping' which provides the trainer with a map on which to plot critical points in the consultation for reflection and future use. A rating scale is also provided to grade the achievement of each task.
- Neighbour (1987) offers five checkpoints to guide the discussion with patients. These highlight tasks as well as specific skills needed in the consultation and the format can be used to assess the learner's awareness of the issues addressed.
- The Calgary–Cambridge Observation Guides (Kurtz and Silverman, 1996; Kurtz *et al.*, 2003) outline the content of a communication skills curriculum based on research and theory and which aid doctor–patient communication as well as structuring the consultation. The Guides have a summary of communication skills which serve as an aide-mémoire and can be used by teachers and learners.
- The SEGUE (set the stage; elicit the information; give information; understand the patient's perspective; end the encounter) framework (Makoul, 1995, 2001) serves as a prompt of the five areas on which to focus during the consultation.

The models share the same theme of listening to the patient and getting their view of the manifestation of the issue under discussion. Of these models the Calgary–Cambridge Observation Guides and the SEGUE ones are frequently used in training and teaching sessions of healthcare professionals. An example of the structure and subdivisions showing the similarities of these two models is outlined in *Table 5.2.*

**Table 5.2** Calgary–Cambridge and SEGUE models of consultation showing two divisions and subdivisions

| Model | Structure of consultation proposed by model | Subdivisions |
|---|---|---|
| Calgary–Cambridge Observation Guides (Kurtz and Silverman, 1996) | Initiating the session includes: (i) preparation; (ii) establishing initial rapport; (iii) identifying the reasons for the consultation | Greeting<br>Establishing initial rapport e.g. demonstrates interest, concern and respect for the patient as a person (here and throughout the interview)<br>Identifying the reasons for the consultation, e.g. listening to the patient's opening statement; checks and confirms list of problems |
| | Gathering information includes: (i) biomedical perspective; (ii) the patient's perspective; (iii) background information | Exploration of the patient's problems to ascertain:<br>The patient's perspective, e.g. encourage patient to tell their story of the problem, when it started and reasons for presenting now<br>Background information – context of the issue: uses open-ended questions and closed questions as appropriate<br>Providing structure to the consultation, e.g. progressing from one section to another using transitional statements; attends to timing and keeping interview focused on task |
| The SEGUE framework (Makoul, 2001) | Set the stage includes: (i) greet the patient appropriately; (ii) establish reason for visit; (iii) outline agenda for visit; (iv) privacy | Greet the patient appropriately<br>Establish the reason for the visit<br>Outline agenda for the visit ('anything else?')<br>Make a personal connection during the visit<br>Maintain patient's privacy, e.g. volume of speech; closed door |
| | Elicit information includes: (I) patient's view of problem; (ii) physical factors; (iii) psychological factors; (iv) antecedent treatments, e.g. prior visit, self care; (vi) effect on patient's life | Elicit patient's view of health problem/ and or progress<br>Explore physical/physiological factors<br>Explore psychological factors<br>Discuss antecedent treatments (including self-care)<br>Discuss how patient's life is affected<br>Discuss lifestyle issues/prevention strategies<br>Avoid directive/leading questions<br>Give patient opportunity/time to talk without interruption<br>Listen. Give patient undivided attention<br>Check/clarify information |

In a real live encounter with patients, the logical structure of the consultation process rarely follows the proposed pattern of the models, but most of the stages are addressed, including the real reason why the visit was made in the first place. Often this is revealed at the end of the consultation and just before the patient leaves the consultation area!

The history-taking component inevitably overlaps with those of the consultation process. Shah (2005) suggests having a guide to undertake the history of the presenting problem, although this may not follow the linear structure he proposes in *Figure 5.1*.

The quality of the doctor–patient communication is a key determinant of whether or not patients' expectations will be met and optimum outcomes achieved. Maguire and Pitceathly (2002) have shown that effective communication leads to patient satisfaction and understanding of their problems, investigation and treatment; it also accounts for improvement in concordance and reduction of stress and depression. Poor communication is often cited when disputes about healthcare arise. Studies have found that patients placed high ratings on interpersonal communication (Wensing *et al.*, 1998), technical competence, listening and informing, taking account of patients' preferences and involving patients in decisions (Coulter and Fitzpatrick, 2000; Jenkins *et al.*, 2002). Patients' preferences regarding the style of communication they would like from healthcare professionals will depend on a variety of factors, including the type and severity of their problem.

Listening and talking to patients are among the basic skills required of the healthcare professional. Yet effectively listening and communicating with patients can be an area of difficulty for some healthcare professionals, but they must be mastered as they are crucial to the consultation process. Consultation skills refer to a range of behaviours that are required during the patient encounter. For example, in *Table 5.3*, the Calgary–Cambridge Observation Guides (Kurtz and Silverman, 1996) approach to consultation skills for 'Identifying the reason for the consultation' and 'Gathering information' shows a breakdown of the variety of behaviours and activities that are required to meet this subcomponent and component, respectively. These procedures may prove challenging for some non-medical prescribers given the short time allowed for some consultations. The next section reflects on the issues relating to consultation with non-medical prescribers.

## Consultation with non-medical prescribers

The UK literature on non-medical prescribers (other than for nurses) and their consultation skills is sparse, mainly because the concept of prescribing by professions allied to medicine is new. However, literature on pharmacist consultation skills is available (Morrow, 1997; Hargie *et al.*, 2000; Abdel Tawab *et al.*, 2005; Greenwood *et al.*, 2006). These studies mainly centre on

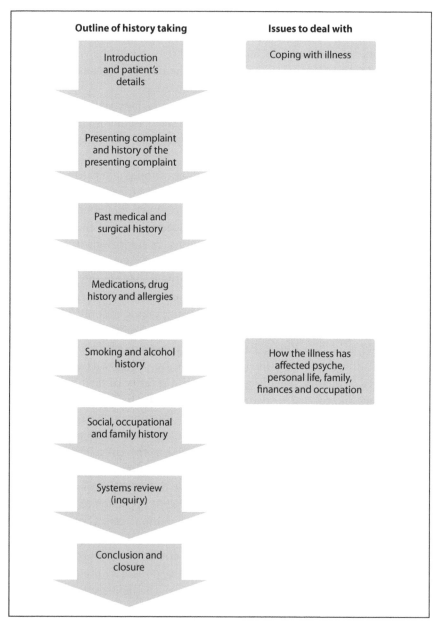

**Outline of history taking**          **Issues to deal with**

Introduction and patient's details

Coping with illness

Presenting complaint and history of the presenting complaint

Past medical and surgical history

Medications, drug history and allergies

Smoking and alcohol history

How the illness has affected psyche, personal life, family, finances and occupation

Social, occupational and family history

Systems review (inquiry)

Conclusion and closure

**Figure 5.1** Components in taking a medical history. Modified from Shah (2005) with kind permission of the BMJ Publishing Group.

the effectiveness of pharmacists' input into the care of patients, the effectiveness of patient–pharmacist consultation and differences between consultation about over-the-counter medicine and prescription medicines. Abdel Tawab *et al.* (2005) have developed a medication-related consultation framework (MRCF) for use with pharmacists. The framework consists of five main

**Table 5.3** Consultation skills and history taking: identifying reasons for consultation and gathering information

| Model | Component of consultation | Behaviours and activities required |
|---|---|---|
| Calgary–Cambridge Observation Guides (Kurtz and Silverman, 1996) | Initiating the session: *subcomponent:* Identifying reasons for the consultation | Identifies problems with appropriate opening question<br>Listens without interrupting<br>Confirms list and screens for other problems early<br>Negotiate agenda |
| | Gathering information | Encourages patient to tell story, in own words, clarifying reason for attending now<br>Uses open and closed question technique<br>Listens attentively – do not allow yourself to be distracted by other things or people<br>Facilitates – verbal and non-verbal responses, use of silence, repetition, etc.<br>Picks up verbal and non-verbal cues<br>Clarifies patient understanding – be patient with those who are not articulate<br>Periodically summarises – reflect on what is being said rather than who is saying it<br>Uses concise, easily understood, jargon-free statements<br>Establishes dates and sequence of events<br>Ideas, concerns, expectations<br>Encourages patient to express feelings<br>Avoid thinking about what you want to say next |

Calgary–Cambridge Observation Guides (Kurtz and Silverman, 1996).

sections: (1) introduction, (2) data collection and problem identification; (3) action and solution; (4) closing and (5) consultation behaviours. Each section has a number of competencies of which there are 46 in total. For example, the Introduction section consists of six competencies of which 'Discusses purpose and structure of the consultation' is one. This framework is still in its infancy and research is needed on its validity, reliability and practicality. These issues are explored in the next section in relation to diagnostics and screening.

## Diagnostics and screening

As healthcare becomes more sophisticated, more conditions are likely to be identified; it is anticipated that more tests will be developed to meet these needs. Some of these development tests may be diagnostic or screening ones. Diagnostic tests serve two different functions: (1) they are used to confirm that a patient has a particular disease; or (2) they are used to exclude that the patient has a particular disease. The same test does not serve both purposes equally well. Confirmation of a diagnosis requires that the test results are reliable; exclusion of diagnosis requires that negative results are reliable (Wulff and Gøtzsche, 2000).

The diagnostic outcome can be one of four possibilities:

1 **True positive** – this result comes about when an abnormality has been detected and the laboratory test confirms this

2 **True negative** – when there is no evidence of abnormality and the various tests indicate this

3 **False positive** – the diagnosing of a normal condition as abnormal (in other words, a false alarm)

4 **False negative** is the opposite of false positive (a miss or misinterpretation of the results).

These false and negative terms are another way of expressing conditional probabilities. 'A conditional probability is the probability of an event occurring given that another has already taken place' (Schwartz and Griffin, 1986: 47). Joint probabilities, on the other hand, refer to the probability of two conditions occurring simultaneously. In clinical diagnosis, doctors are interested in knowing the conditional probability of normal and abnormal diagnoses given certain test results. In other words, a true positive result is the conditional probability of an abnormal diagnosis when the patient's condition is abnormal.

Screening is a public health service which puts the benefits of reduced mortality and morbidity as too important to be left to the individual to decide whether or not they should participate (Marteau and Kinmonth, 2002). It is a service which is offered to individuals of a defined population who (1) may be asymptomatic of a disease but who may have early disease, (2) are at risk of a disease, or (3) may be already affected by a disease or its complications. Screening is one option for diagnosis; depending on the patient's condition, they can be referred for further testing or examination to assist the healthcare professional with diagnosis. Criteria for the validity, effectiveness and appropriateness of screening were developed by Wilson and Jungner (1968) but has extended to include risk factors such as blood pressure, cholesterol and susceptibility (e.g. HIV status). The National Screening Committee criteria for screening is based on Wilson and Jungner's four criteria:

1 **Knowledge of the disease**: The disease should be serious enough to warrant large scale screening and the natural course of the disease should be adequately understood.

2 **Knowledge of the test:** The test should be acceptable to the population.

3 **Treatment for the disease:** Accepted treatment should be available for patients with the disease and treatment before symptoms develop should be more beneficial in reducing mortality and morbidity than later treatment.

4 **Cost implications:** The costs of finding cases (including diagnosis and treatment of patients diagnosed with the disease) should outweigh possible expenditures on medical care as a whole.

In essence, the implication of screening tests is that they should do more good than harm. However, the National Screening Committee (NSC) (2000: 2) say that patients should be made aware of the possible risks when undergoing screening:

> *There is a responsibility to ensure that those who accept an invitation [to screening] do so on the basis of informed choice and appreciate that in accepting an invitation or participating in a programme to reduce their risk of a disease there is a risk of an adverse outcome.*

Nonetheless, the underlying issue for healthcare professionals is one of making a correct decision.

## The rationale for correct decision making

The rationale for correct decision making lies in the effective treatment of patients once a diagnosis has been made. Effective treatment of patients depends on the practitioner's consulting and history-taking skills, leading to a correct diagnosis. Fowler (1997) believes that skill in diagnosis depends on the practitioner's knowledge of what happens rather than why issues arise. According to Fowler, the practitioner should be aware of the different modes of onset of symptoms, for example, sudden, rapid, slow and insidious onset of illness so that the mode is incorporated into the practitioner's cognition during the decision-making process. The decision-making process should incorporate research evidence (if available), the patient's views and beliefs and enough information to assist the patient to make informed choices about their healthcare. Thus, the healthcare practitioner must decide which data are the most reliable, accurate and representative of true evidence rather than speculation.

## Focus on practice and implementation

The expansion of non-medical prescribing means that practitioners will require a solid grounding in the principles of therapeutic as well as scientific knowledge about drug interaction (Maxwell and Walley, 2003). This is reinforced by Avery and Pringle's (2005) view that prescribing is one of the most powerful tools that health professionals can use in tackling disease. Conversely, it can also cause significant morbidity and mortality (Maxwell and Walley, 2003). Over a decade ago, Barber (1995) elucidated the case for 'good prescribing' citing four main aims that the 'good prescriber' should aim to achieve when making the decision to prescribe and when monitoring the drug. The aims are: to maximise effectiveness, minimise risks, minimise costs, and respect the patient's choices. In today's climate, Primary Care Trusts face added challenges of treating some patients' conditions with new and very expensive drugs, providing healthcare services for their population, balancing conflicts while operating within their financial resource allocation.

Current courses training non-medical prescribers must be of an appropriate length to equip them for their practice. It is also important that they know how errors occur in practice and incorporate these principles in the assessment of risk management. It is also essential that continuing professional development in the form of further training opportunities, including work-based educational support and mentorship, are in place to assist prescribers in their work. This requires financial and organisational support as well as access to technology. Avery and Pringle (2005) extend this view by suggesting that robust clinical governance arrangements should be in place to identify prescribers – medical and non-medical – who exceed their competency.

While the Government advocates new ways of working to maximise and liberate the potential of all healthcare professionals, this involves rigorous management and monitoring practice as well as a change in mindset among and within multiprofessionals. Medical practitioners who act as designated medical practitioners in the education, mentoring and assessing of other healthcare professionals need to be supported to prepare and undertake these activities. This involves joint working with the organisation and higher education institutions to ensure agreed standards are maintained and the quality of teaching and assessing are robust. With these safeguards in place, the implications for non-medical prescribing include the following:

- There are increased opportunities for collaboration due to prescriptive authority.
- The prescriber is seen as a resource for medication in specific areas.
- The prescriptive authority is likely to encourage networking with other professions.
- The prescriptive authority influences the patient journey.
- There is increased satisfaction with care from both the perspective of both patient and professional.

Nonetheless, the new ways of working attract errors and pitfalls of which the prescriber and decision maker should be aware, some of which are outlined in the next section.

## Errors and pitfalls to avoid

Russo and Schoemaker (1991) succinctly sum up ten common errors to avoid in the decision-making process:

1 Plunging-in: a situation where decision makers begin to gather information and make decisions without first considering the wider picture.
2 Frame blindness: in which a mental framework of the issues has been formed without looking at all the options or important points.
3 Lack of frame control: a one-sided view of the problem or being unduly influenced by the perspective of others.
4 Overconfidence in one's judgement: results from a failure to collect information from all angles because of confidence in one's own views.
5 Short-sighted shortcuts: an over-reliance on 'rules of thumb', an unshakeable belief in one's intuition, or too much focus on easily available data.
6 Shooting from the hip: results from a belief that all the relevant information can be mentally retained without resort to a systematic procedure for the final decision.
7 Group failure: this arises from a failure on the part of the facilitator to manage the group decision process and believing that 'well-placed' individuals will have the right answers.
8 Fooling yourself about feedback: demonstrates a failure to learn from past experience.
9 Not keeping track: failing to keep systematic records of past results of decisions and a failure to analyse these results and highlight the pertinent issues.
10 Failure to audit one's decision process: failure to examine the decision-making process in a way that enhances understanding of past behaviour.

## Conclusions

Non-medical prescribing provides the opportunity for improvement in patient care, quicker access to health professionals and provides choice for them. It also increases collaboration between health professionals. However, vigorous and robust governance procedures should be in place where non-medical prescribers operate. Ongoing work-based training and support will be needed which will involve budgeting implications for the organisation. Thus, non-medical prescribing is not a cheap or easy option.

## Further reading

Abdel Tawab R, Davies JG, Horne R and James DH (2005). Evaluating pharmaceutical consultations: a validation of the medical-related consultation framework (MRCF). *Int J Pharm Pract* 13 (suppl): R27.

Brookes D. and Smith A (2006). *Non-Medical Prescribing in Healthcare Practice: A toolkit for students and practitioners.* Basingstoke: Palgrave Macmillan.

Coulter A and Fitzpatrick R (2000). The patient's perspective regarding appropriate health care. In: Albrecht GL, Fitzpatrick R and Scrimshaw RC (eds) *The Handbook of Social Studies in Health and Medicine.* London: SAGE.

Hargie ODW, Murrow NC and Woodman C (2000). Pharmacists' evaluation of key communication skills in practice. *Patient Educ Couns* 39: 61–70.

Sackett DL, Rosenberg W, Gray JA, Haynes RB and Richardson WS (1996). Evidence-based medicine: what it is and what it isn't. *BMJ* 312: 71–72.

## References

Abdel Tawab R, Davies JG, Horne R and James DH (2005). Evaluating pharmaceutical consultations: a validation of the medical-related consultation framework (MRCF). *Int J Pharm Pract* 13 (suppl): R27.

Avery AJ and Pringle M (2005). Extended prescribing by UK nurses and pharmacists. *BMJ* 331: 1154–1155.

Balint M (1957). *The Doctor, His Patient and the Illness.* London: Pitman Medical.

Barber N (1995). What constitutes good prescribing? *BMJ* 310: 923–925.

Brunswik E (1952). *The Conceptual Framework of Psychology.* Chicago: University of Chicago.

Byrne P and Long BEL (1976). *Doctors Talking to Patients.* London: HMSO.

Coulter A and Fitzpatrick R (2000). The patient's perspective regarding appropriate health care. In: Albrecht GL, Fitzpatrick R and Scrimshaw RC (eds) *The Handbook of Social Studies in Health and Medicine.* London: SAGE.

Doherty ME and Kurz EM (1996). Social judgement theory. In: Doherty M (ed.) *Thinking and Reasoning.* Exeter: Psychology Press, pp. 109–140.

Ericsson KA and Simon HA (1993). *Protocol Analysis: Verbal Reports as Data.* Cambridge, MA: MIT Press.

Fowler PBS (1997). Evidenced-based diagnosis. *J Eval Clin Pract* 3: 153–159.

Greenwood K, Howe A and Holland R (2006). The use of consultation skills assessment tool in pharmacist–patient consultations. *Int J Pharm Pract* 14: 277–282.

Hamm RM (1988). Clinical intuition and clinical analysis: expertise and the cognitive continuum. In: Dowie J and Elstein A (eds) *Professional Judgement: A reader in clinical decision making.* Cambridge: Cambridge University Press.

Hammond KR (1978). Towards increasing competence of thought in public policy formation. In: Hammond KR (ed.) *Judgement and Decision in Public Policy Formation.* Boulder CO: Westview Press, pp. 11–32.

Hargie ODW, Murrow NC and Woodman C (2000). Pharmacists' evaluation of key communication skills in practice. *Patient Educ Couns* 39: 61–70.

Jenkins L, Barber N, Bradley CP and Stevenson FA (2002). Consultations do not have to be longer. *BMJ* 325: 388.

Kahneman D, Slovic P and Tversky A (eds) (1982). *Judgement under Uncertainty: Heuristics and Biases.* Cambridge: Cambridge University Press.

Kurtz S and Silverman J (1996). The Calgary–Cambridge observation guides: an aid to defining the curriculum and organising the teaching in communication and training programmes. *Med Educ* 30: 83–89.

Kurtz S, Silverman J and Draper J (2003). Marrying content and process in clinical method teaching: enhancing the Calgary–Cambridge Guides. *Acad Med* 78: 802–809.

Maguire P and Pitceathly C (2002). Key communication skills and how to acquire them. *BMJ* 325: 697–700.

Makoul G (1995). *SEGUE: a framework for teaching and evaluating communication in medical encounters.* San Francisco: Division 1 of the American Educational Research Association.

Makoul G (2001). The SEGUE framework for teaching and assessing communication skills. *Patient Educ Couns* 45: 23–34.

Marteau TM and Kinmonth AL (2002). Screening for cardiovascular risk: public health imperative or a matter for individual informed choice? *BMJ* 325: 78–80.

Maxwell SRJ and Walley T (2003). Teaching prescribing and therapeutics. *Br J Clin Pharmacol* 55: 496–503.

Maxwell SRJ, Walley T and Ferner RE (2002). Using drugs safely. *BMJ* 324: 930–931.

Morrow D (1997). Improving consultations between health-care professionals and older clients: implications for pharmacists. *Int J Aging Hum Dev* 44: 47–72.

Neighbour R (1987). *The Inner Consultation.* Lancaster: MTO Press.

Newell A and Simon HA (1972). *Human Problem Solving.* Englewood Cliffs, NJ: Prentice Hall.

Offredy M (2002). Decision making in primary care: outcomes from a study using patient scenarios. *J Adv Nurs* 40(5): 532–541.

Offredy M, Kendall S and Goodman C (2008). The use of cognitive continuum theory and patient scenarios to explore nurse prescribers' pharmacological knowledge and decision making. *Int J Nurs Stud* 45: 855–868.

Pendelton D, Schofield T, Tate P and Havelock P (1984). *The Consultation: An approach to learning and teaching.* Oxford: Oxford University Press.

Pendelton D, Schofield T, Tate P and Havelock P (2003). *The New Consultation.* Oxford: Oxford University Press.

Raiffa H (1970). *Decision Analysis: Introductory lectures on choices under uncertainty. Reading*, MA: Addison-Wesley.

Russo EJ and Schoemaker PJH (1991). *Confident Decision Making.* London: Piatkus Books.

Sackett DL, Rosenberg W, Gray JA, Haynes RB and Richardson WS (1996). Evidence-based medicine: what it is and what it isn't. *BMJ* 312: 71–72.

Schwartz S and Griffin T (1986) *Medical Thinking: The psychology of medical judgement and decision making.* New York: Springer-Verlag.

Shah N (2005). Taking a history: introduction and the presenting complaint. *Student BMJ* 13: 309–352.

Tanner CA, Padrick K, Westfall UE and Putzier DJ (1987). Diagnostic reasoning strategies of nurses and nursing students. *Nurs Res* 36: 358–363.

Weinstein MC and Fineberg HV (1980). *Clinical Decision Analysis.* Philadelphia: WB Saunders.

Wensing M, Jung HP, Mainz J, Olesen F and Grol R (1998). A systematic review of the literature on patient prioroities for general practice care. Part 1: description of the reseach domain. *Soc Sci Med* 47: 1573–1588.

Wilson JMG and Jungner G (1968). *Principles and Practice for Screening Disease.* Geneva: World Health Organization.

Wulff HR and Gøtzsche PC (2000). *Rational Diagnosis and Treatment: Evidence-based clinical decision making*, 3rd edn. Oxford: Blackwell Science.

# 6

# Prescribing in diabetes

*Alan Sinclair*

---

**Key learning points:**

- Overview of the disease state
- Key issues for prescribing in this clinical area
- Overview of knowledge and skills for safe and effective prescribing
- Clinical case studies to demonstrate issues in non-medical prescribing.

---

## Introduction and background

In the UK there are nearly 2 million people with diagnosed diabetes and possibly as many as a million people with undiagnosed diabetes. This creates a tremendous personal health burden and is associated with significant healthcare expenditure in the National Health Service (NHS). Factors such as the ageing of the population, increasing levels of obesity and higher prevalence rates in Asian and Afro-Caribbean people contribute to these changes (Diabetes UK, 2004).

Diabetes is a chronic disease which can be associated with disabling vascular complications, including renal disease and visual loss. Cardiovascular disease is a major cause of reduced survival. At the time of diagnosis as many as half of the people with diabetes may have evidence of complications and so early detection is important.

Lifestyle changes and appropriate treatment regimens coupled with empowering people with diabetes to self-care can help to reduce this health burden and improve quality of life and outcomes. Effective use of non-medical prescribing can assist in meeting the challenge of diabetes.

It was the National Service Framework (NSF) for Diabetes (Department of Health, 2001) which recognised that 'diabetes is a chronic life-long condition that impacts upon almost every aspect of life. Living with diabetes is not easy. Medication is usually self-administered.' It is not surprising that effective diabetes care may involve a multidisciplinary team including specialist nurses, medics, dieticians, podiatrists, optometrists, pharmacists and psychologists. Global clinical care of people with diabetes may involve multiple medications, such as glucose-lowering medicines and therapies which lower blood pressure or blood lipids, and reduce the likelihood of thromboembolism and other vascular complications of diabetes.

This chapter will focus on the clinical area of diabetes and explore the potential benefits and limitations of a non-medical prescribing programme based on the Department of Health's three criteria justifying this approach, that is:

1 improves patients' quick access to medicines
2 improves access to care services
3 allows more efficient use of nurses' and other health professionals' skills.

The discussion will relate predominantly to nurse and pharmacy prescribing, although in selected examples other health professionals could be identified to participate in non-medical prescribing (e.g. optometrists or physiotherapists). There will be no attempt to discuss individually each of the three categories of non-medical prescribing, namely nurse independent prescribers, the pharmacist independent prescriber, and supplementary prescribing by nurses, pharmacists and other allied health professionals. The latter prescribing activities are usually within set clinical management plans.

Previous formularies were invariably too resource intensive to maintain, often too complex to use and did not provide adequate prescribing information in all settings. Indeed, progress was only made with non-medical prescribing when the Committee on Safety of Medicines (CSM) recently considered responses to several consultations and concluded that suitably trained and qualified nurses and pharmacists should be able to prescribe any licensed medicine for any medical condition, within their own competence.

The Government's intention is that by extending prescribing responsibilities to healthcare professionals other than doctors and dentists, some key objectives of the NHS plan can be achieved:

1 The needs of local health economies are being addressed by health professionals taking on extended roles and responsibilities.
2 More flexible services can be offered and there is an increased opportunity to complete episodes of care for those groups where usual access to care is compromised or patients are particularly vulnerable.

Detailed comments about creating 'patient group directions' for nurses and pharmacists is also outside the scope of this chapter, but within NHS settings these are often a vehicle for ensuring safe and reliable non-medical prescribing by those with the appropriate knowledge/skills mix.

## Description of key issues

Work commissioned by Skills for Health on behalf of the Diabetes Workforce Executive Group at the Department of Health has reported its early findings of review in this area (Skills for Health, 2006). Modern diabetes healthcare is a multiprofessional process with several key individual professions having the ability to acquire the appropriate knowledge, skills and attitudes to undertake effective diabetes care. However, initial findings suggested that some concerns would need to be addressed:

- Is sufficient 'capacity' available within current diabetes nursing services to enable diabetes specialist nurses (DSNs) to undertake training in supplementary prescribing?
- Can clinical management plans for each patient be developed in reasonable time frames?
- How do we ensure clarity in the way patients are managed by both a specialist diabetes team and a diabetes team in primary care?
- Are some aspects of the training entirely relevant to non-medical prescribing?

## Brief summary of the knowledge areas and skills required for safe prescribing

The knowledge areas required can be summarised as:

- the pathophysiology of diabetes mellitus and its classification into the two major types, type 1 and type 2; the relationship to the metabolic syndrome
- the importance of lifestyle modifications and the benefits of regular exercise
- the special features of diabetes in children, young people, the elderly and pregnancy
- the spectrum of both microvascular and macrovascular complications
- general principles of the clinical pharmacology of oral hypoglycaemic agents and insulin, including knowledge of adverse drug reactions and other side-effects (e.g. hypoglycaemia)
- knowledge of other related treatment areas: lipid lowering, antihypertensive medication, antiplatelet therapy.

A framework for denoting the competencies and skills required of nurse and pharmacist prescribers is being developed by the National Prescribing Centre. Within diabetes care, additional skills required for safe and effective non-medical prescribing practice are:

- working familiarity with basic nutritional planning and lifestyle modification practices

- consultation skills and appreciation of the need to empower people with diabetes to diabetes self-manage
- self-blood glucose monitoring (SBGM) and its interpretation
- diagnostic skills and some skills in differential diagnostics; skills in interpreting laboratory data
- the use of oral hypoglycaemic agents and insulin within the scope of a clinical management plan
- how to adjust dosage in the light of symptom profiles and blood glucose measures and HbA1c levels
- how to consider the introduction of additional glucose-lowering therapy and adjunctive therapy with lipid-lowering agents, blood-pressure-lowering therapy and antiplatelet agents
- how to balance the adverse effects of treatment with the likely benefits in different patient categories.

## Prescribing scenarios – diabetes

### Case study 1

A 55-year-old business man was seen with resistant balanitis but otherwise was well. His BMI was 32. A random glucose level was 14.4 mmol/L.

**1 What do the signs and symptoms indicate?**
Difficult to treat or recurrent balanitis might suggest diabetes but the raised random glucose is significant. He is obese, which has increased the risk of diabetes.

**2 What is the prescribing issue?**
He requires advice and support to engage in an intensive lifestyle management plan. The prescriber would need to decide if an oral agent should also be commenced.

**3 How would you deal with this?**
Ask for a fasting glucose level and an HbA1c. If the fasting glucose level is >7.0 mmol/L and taken together with his symptoms and previous elevated glucose level, this patient has diabetes. A raised HbA1c would provide additional support for this diagnosis. Additional laboratory tests should be considered.

In this instance, I would recommend a weight loss programme and intensive lifestyle modification for 6–8 weeks with review. Patient to return early if symptoms continue. Access to a community dietician and diabetes specialist nurse would complement this programme. Continuation of antifungal treatment (if previously prescribed) may be necessary depending on the advice of the GP.

**4 What are the benefits to the patient?**
Symptom improvement and weight loss. Improvement in glucose level. Introduction of new lifestyle. May be able to avoid drug therapy at this stage.

## Case study 2

A 39-year-old woman taking a twice-daily insulin regimen for type 1 diabetes is complaining of disturbed sleep, feeling sweaty when she wakes, and her recent HbA1c was 7.5%.

**1 What do the signs and symptoms indicate?**
Episodes of hypoglycaemia occurring at night combined with poor glycaemic control.

**2 What is the prescribing issue?**
Change in the dosage of the current insulin regimen or switching to a basal-bolus regimen?

**3 How would you deal with this?**
Review dietary plan and evening snacks. Review insulin administration skills. Ensure that poor control is not due to an infection (e.g. urinary infection).

Switch to a basal-bolus regimen giving greater flexibility and likelihood of achieving adequate glycaemic levels. Monitor 'hypos' and ask for SBGM information from the patient. Adjust the doses of insulin accordingly.

**4 What are the benefits to the patient?**
Greater flexibility with meals and timings of insulin injections. Reduce risk of hypoglycaemia. Improved glycaemic control aiming for 7% or lower.

## Case study 3

A 80-year-old woman has type 2 diabetes and is on maximum doses of metformin and gliclazide. Her HbA1c is 8.6%. She feels generally tired and has had several falls recently. Her vision has worsened in the previous 12 months.

**1 What do the signs and symptoms indicate?**
Poor glycaemic control producing lethargy and worse vision which has increased the risk of falling.

**2 What is the prescribing issue?**
Should a third oral agent be added, such as a thiazolidinedione (say pioglitazone) or should insulin be considered?

**3 How would you deal with this?**
Check adherence to therapy and assess reading ability and distance vision using a Snellan chart. Refer to optician if necessary. Check her balance by asking the patient to rise from a chair unaided, walk a few steps, and return

to the chair, and sit. Suggest to the patient that she visits an optometrist for a vision and eye check-up.

If mentally competent and generally fit otherwise, would suggest a trial of insulin to achieve better glycaemic control in a shorter period of time. Aim for a HbA1c <7.5%, stop gliclazide, and remain on metformin. Would need to involve GP in discussions about initiation of insulin and where and how it should take place.

If the patient is rather frail and lacks support at home, the risk of hypoglycaemia may be too high and adding in a third oral agent might be more appropriate. Advise more frequent blood glucose monitoring by patient or district nurse.

### 4 What are the benefits to the patient?
Improved glucose control and less risk of metabolic decompensation. Vision may improve if glucose improves and falls risk may be less.

## Case study 4

A 59-year-old man has had type 2 diabetes for 9 years and is treated by diet and metformin. His HbA1c is 8.3%. He feels relatively well but has started to complain of disturbed sleep due to painful feet. He describes these symptoms as 'tingling' and occasionally 'burning'. He only notices this at night-time and gets some relief from getting up and walking about. These symptoms appear to be getting worse.

### 1 What do the signs and symptoms indicate?
He may be developing signs of small-fibre neuropathy which is a form of distal sensorimotor polyneuropathy. Long-standing poor glycaemic control may contribute to this.

### 2 What is the prescribing issue?
A detailed history should distinguish between pain of neuropathic origin and that of vascular origin. In some cases, pain may be self-limiting with no obvious explanation. Some patients may have already taken an over-the-counter analgesic.

The range of treatments for neuropathic pain range from standard analgesics (e.g non-steroidal anti-inflammatory drugs), to topical application of capsaicin, a drug which depletes substance P. Antidepressant and anticonvulsant therapies are also employed.

### 3 How would you deal with this?
If symptoms are inconclusive and less urgent, and the patient has no history of vascular-like problems (e.g. discolouration of toes, cramps in the back of the leg when walking – 'intermittent claudication' or obvious heart disease) you could consider standard analgesics initially for several weeks, and ask

the patient to examine his feet daily to look for any injury. You can get hold of pain assessment charts which can sometimes help to monitor the pain.

If symptoms continue, the patient requires referral for full examination (peripheral nervous system, leg pulses, blood pressure, etc.) since further investigation and more specific neuropathic pain relief may be required.

The usual programme to maintain a healthy lifestyle and improve glycaemic control is necessary.

### 4 What are the benefits to the patient?

Painful feet can influence quality of life dramatically and can lead to further damaged feet and even disability. The detection of neuropathy is important since although diabetes is likely to be the cause, other forms of neuropathy can occur and another systemic disorder may be present.

This is also an opportunity for the non-medical prescriber to educate the patient about foot protection and wearing suitable footwear. Referral to a podiatrist can also be suggested if necessary.

## Case study 5

A 74-year-old woman has had type 2 diabetes for 4 years and is treated by diet and gliclazide. She is involved in diabetes self-management and her twice-daily capillary glucose levels range from 5 to 9 mmol/L and her HbA1c is 7.4%.

She has complained of frequency of micturition for the last 7 weeks but has no other symptoms apart from an intermittent mild backache. These symptoms are beginning to affect her social life and she is reluctant to go out for long periods of time unless she knows that she has ready access to toilet facilities.

### 1 What do the signs and symptoms indicate?

This patient may have an untreated urinary tract infection with some possible upper renal tract involvement.

### 2. What is the prescribing issue?

Whilst poor glycaemic control can cause polyuria (passing large volumes of urine) this is not the case here. Her HbA1c is not too high and further history denotes that she passes only small amounts frequently.

She is likely to require a course of antibiotics (at least 7 days) but her urine has to be tested for bacteriuria before commencing the course. In addition, any further symptoms of backache require immediate referral to a doctor to exclude the presence of pyelonephritis.

Choosing the right antibiotic in patients with diabetes and uncomplicated urine infections can sometimes be problematical. In this case, trimethoprim is likely to undertreat and so either a quinolone (e.g. ciprofloxacin) or a third-generation cephalosporin may be required.

## 3 How would you deal with this?

If the patient is relatively well and the symptoms of backache are minor and not troublesome, it may be worth considering a course of antibiotic treatment. A urine dipstick test to look for protein, blood or white cells would provide additional evidence of infection but a properly obtained mid-stream urine (MSU) sample must be sent to the hospital laboratory. The patient should be asked about symptoms of vaginal irritation as candidiasis can mimic these symptoms.

A 7-day course of treatment should be offered while waiting for the laboratory confirmation. The patient should be advised to drink plenty of fluids and report to her GP if she becomes unwell or her symptoms worsen. Admission to hospital and intravenous antibiotic therapy may be necessary in more serious cases.

## 4 What are the benefits to the patient?

Symptoms often improve after about 3 days of treatment but the full course must be taken in most cases.

Untreated urinary infections can lead to pyelonephritis and serious kidney damage. Prompt treatment is essential and a full course of treatment is important. In some cases, where symptoms do not resolve, a fungal infection may be present, requiring a different treatment, or the patient has a bladder or kidney problem requiring further investigation by medical staff.

## Further reading

Department of Health (2006). A guide to implementing nurse and pharmacist independent prescribing within the NHS in England. http://www.dh.gov.uk/assetRoot/04/13/37/47/04133747.pdf

National Institute for Health and Clinical Excellence (NICE) (CG66, May 2008). Diabetes – Type 2. This is an update of the following guidelines: Type 2 Diabetes – retinopathy (Published February 2002). Type 2 Diabetes – renal disease (Published February 2002). Type 2 Diabetes – blood glucose (Published September 2002). Type 2 Diabetes – management of blood pressure and blood lipids (Published October 2002). Type 2 Diabetes – Footcare (first update published January 2004) (As this is recently published, it will not be updated, but parts may be referred to or incorporated into the new guideline.)

## References

Department of Health (2001). National Service Framework for Diabetes: Standards. London: Department of Health.

Diabetes UK (2004). Diabetes in the UK. www.diabetes.org.uk

Skills for Health (2006). A report from the Diabetes Workforce Executive Group: Non-medical Prescribing in Diabetes. Part 1: Early findings. London: Clinical Governance Support Team, National Diabetes Support Team.

# 7

# Prescribing in palliative care

*Jo Noble-Gresty*

**Key learning points:**

- Overview of the management area
- Key issues for prescribing in this clinical area
- Overview of knowledge and skills for safe and effective prescribing
- Clinical case studies to demonstrate issues in non-medical prescribing.

## Introduction and background

*Palliative care is the approach that improves the quality of life of patients and their families facing the problems associated with life-threatening illness, through the prevention and relief of suffering by means of early identification and impeccable assessment and treatment of pain and other problems, physical, psychosocial and spiritual. (World Health Organization, 2005)*

The driving force behind palliative care is the desire to transform dying.

While the majority of palliative care patients have advanced cancer, often with multiple sites of metastases, other life-limiting illnesses are also seen; the end-stage neurological diseases (e.g. motor neurone disease, multiple sclerosis, multi-system atrophy, Parkinson's disease), end-stage cardiac, hepatic, renal and respiratory disease and HIV/AIDs.

This chapter will focus on the following key learning points:

- familiarity with symptoms and their treatments
- familiarity with drugs prescribed
- application of assessment skills
- attention to detail for the individual patient
- liability for prescribing drugs off-licence.

Cancer is a major cause of morbidity in the UK. Each year more than 250 000 people are newly diagnosed with cancer, with breast, lung, colorectal and prostate accounting for over half of all new cases. Cancer predominantly occurs in older people, with 64% of cases diagnosed in people aged 65 and over, while 10% of all cancer cases are in the 25–50 age group.

One in four (26%) of all deaths in the UK are caused by cancer and nearly one in five (22%) of all cancer deaths are from lung cancer. Colorectal is the second most common cause of cancer death (10%) and breast cancer the third (8%). One third of all deaths from cancer are linked to tobacco smoking; this includes 88% of lung cancer deaths.

About 76% of cancer deaths occur in people aged 65 years and over. In people under 75 years, deaths from cancer outnumber deaths from disease of the circulatory system, including heart disease and stroke and the respiratory system combined (figures for 2005 from Cancer Research UK).

Specialist palliative care is delivered by hospital palliative care teams, specialist palliative care units within hospitals or hospices and homecare teams within primary care (*Table 7.1*)

Patients are referred to the specialist palliative care service for:

- symptom control
- emotional, psychological and spiritual support
- social and financial advice
- carer support
- assessment for hospice admission
- terminal care.

The holistic approach taken in palliative care acknowledges that suffering is more than physical distress and recognises that patients require a combination of physical, psychological, social and spiritual care. Consequently a

**Table 7.1** Provision of specialist palliative care services in England, Wales and Northern Ireland

| | |
|---|---|
| Specialist inpatient units | 193 providing 2774 beds (20% NHS) |
| Homecare services | 295 |
| Hospital-based services | 314 |
| Day care services | 234 |
| Bereavement support services | 314 |
| From National Council for Palliative Care, January 2006. | |

multidisciplinary approach is required. Doctors, nurses, physiotherapists, occupational therapists, pharmacists, dieticians, speech and language therapists, social workers, chaplains, psychologists, counsellors, complementary therapists, art therapists and music therapists all contribute their expertise to the specialist palliative care team.

## Knowledge and skills required in prescribing in palliative care

The presence of a variety of symptoms can greatly affect the quality of life of the palliative care patient; consequently good symptom control is paramount. Because pharmacological management is often the mainstay of symptom control, the pharmacist has a valuable role to play in the multidisciplinary team. Prescribing in palliative care patients is complex due to multiple symptoms and a changing disease, thus attention to detail is necessary. Continual review is an important factor as drug handling is often affected by disease progression. A good understanding and application of pharmacokinetics is essential, particularly as metabolism and excretion of drugs may be affected by the disease process.

In patients with advanced cancer, the most prevalent and clinically important symptoms are pain, fatigue and anorexia. Other common symptoms are weight loss, insomnia, constipation, depression, nausea and vomiting, dyspnoea and anxiety (Donnelly and Walsh, 1995; Vainio et al., 1996). Familiarity with the possible causes of these symptoms and their treatments is a key requirement.

More than 50% of cancer patients suffer pain, and this is often the most feared symptom. About 64% of patients with metastatic, advanced or terminal disease experience pain, but the highest prevalence, 70%, occurs in head and neck cancer patients (Van den Beuken-van Everdingen et al., 2007). Use of the three-step WHO analgesic ladder (*Figure 7.1*), a validated system for treating chronic cancer pain, achieves satisfactory pain relief in up to 88% of patients (Zech et al., 1995). Familiarity with this framework and the application of its principles is essential to good pain management.

A thorough pain assessment of each pain experienced by the patient should be undertaken and include characteristics, severity, aggravating and relieving factors, history and previous response to treatment. Analgesia should be initiated at the level appropriate for the degree of pain. Opioids are the mainstay of pain management. The use of adjuvant drugs to relieve specific types of pain should also be considered (*Table 7.2*). Analgesics should be taken regularly and access to breakthrough (rescue) analgesia at the appropriate dose should always be available. All patients receiving opioids should receive a softener and stimulant laxative combination to prevent constipation.

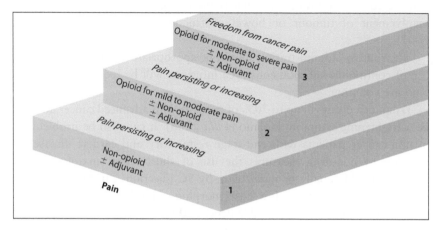

**Figure 7.1** The World Health Organization analgesic ladder.

| Table 7.2 Adjuvant drugs for treating specific pain syndromes ||
| --- | --- |
| NSAIDs | Musculoskeletal pain, bone pain |
| Corticosteroids | Compression by tumour, liver capsule pain |
| Tricyclic antidepressants | Neuropathic pain |
| Anticonvulsants | Neuropathic pain |
| NMDA-receptor channel blockers | Neuropathic pain |
| Bisphosphonates | Bone pain |
| Smooth muscle relaxants | Visceral distension pain and colic |
| Skeletal muscle relaxants | Muscle spasm |

Nausea and vomiting occurs in up to 60% of patients with advanced cancer and most commonly in those under 65 years, in women and in those with stomach, gynaecological or breast cancer (Baines, 1997). Different causes of nausea and vomiting occur via different pathways and neurotransmitters. Pharmacological management should be based on the likely cause and the pathways involved as there are few data from randomised controlled trials of antiemetics in palliative care patients. Understanding and application of these pharmacological principles is necessary for appropriate and successful symptom resolution.

Metoclopramide for gastric stasis, cyclizine for raised intracranial pressure and haloperidol for biochemical induced nausea and vomiting are all first-line antiemetic drugs. Low-dose levomepromazine, a broad-spectrum agent, is useful when first-line agents fail. Dexamethasone should also be considered as an adjuvant agent where there is primary and secondary brain involvement of tumour or bowel obstruction (Twycross and Wilcock, 2007).

The route of administration should be appropriate for the situation, and use of continuous subcutaneous (SC) infusions will be required in patients who are vomiting.

Dyspnoea occurs in up to 70% of patients with advanced cancer and can be a frightening symptom (Solano *et al.*, 2006). It can also be problematic in non-cancer patients with end-stage respiratory and cardiac disease. In addition to non-drug measures the use of short-acting anxiolytics (e.g. lorazepam sublingually or midazolam by SC injection) can help to reduce the fear while the use of low-dose morphine or other opioids decreases respiratory effort (Twycross and Wilcock, 2001).

The subcutaneous route is the route of choice in palliative care patients when parenteral administration is required. Continuous SC infusions of drugs using portable battery-powered syringe drivers are used to control symptoms when the oral route is no longer appropriate. Combinations of drugs may be used for symptom control in specific situations (e.g. vomiting) as well as for end-of-life care. Knowledge of appropriate drugs, doses, diluents and compatibility is necessary together with the technique for setting up a syringe driver.

Usual combinations include up to three of the following drugs, depending on the symptoms experienced by the patient:

- Analgesic (e.g. morphine, diamorphine, oxycodone, alfentanil*, ketamine*, ketorolac*)
- Antiemetic (e.g. cyclizine*, metoclopramide*, haloperidol*, levomepromazine, ondansetron*)
- Antisecretory (e.g. hyoscine butylbromide*, glycopyrronium*)
- Sedative (e.g. midazolam*, levomepromazine).

*Off-licence route of administration.

## General principles of prescribing in palliative care

The cause(s) of the symptoms must be evaluated, together with the impact of the illness on the patient and family. History of the symptom and previous response to medication should be elicited.

Before starting treatment, an explanation should be given about what is going on and the most appropriate course of action. The goal of treatment, incidence reduction versus complete relief, should be clear.

Management should include correcting the correctable if possible, and considering both non-drug treatment and drug treatment. Safe prescribing is particularly important in palliative care patients where the combination of polypharmacy, debility, co-morbidities, involvement of multi-health professionals and the use of higher risk medications make such patients vulnerable to problems with compliance, undesirable effects and medication errors. A systematic approach with attention to detail should be made, with rationalisation of medication regimens to the minimum:

- Is it possible to stop any of the current medication? (e.g. antihypertensives)
- Is the prescribing appropriate? (e.g. statins)
- Is there any duplication? (e.g. laxatives, antiemetics)
- Can the tablet burden be reduced? (e.g. once or twice daily dosing)
- Is the formulation appropriate? (e.g. where patients have problems swallowing or have feeding tubes, then soluble tablets or liquid formulations should be prescribed. The option of the transdermal or oral transmucosal (buccal or sublingual) routes must also be considered.)

Frequent monitoring of the impact of treatment should be made with a view to optimising doses for symptom relief to maximise benefit and minimise adverse effects and drug interactions.

In order to aid compliance, large containers and non-child-resistant lids should be used for dispensing and labelled with clear instructions of the drug regimen. Consider a specific compliance aid if necessary and if the patient is able to use it. A medication record with the drug name and strength, description, dosing, timings in relation to mealtimes and reason for use is a simple but efficient way of improving compliance.

The importance of accurate documentation cannot be overstated. Any consultations and interventions must be fully documented in the patient's notes.

Up to a quarter of all prescriptions in palliative care are for drugs used off-licence (Atkinson and Kirkham, 1999; Todd and Davies, 1999). There are few randomised controlled clinical trials of symptomatic treatments in advanced disease because of the barriers to conducting such studies in palliative care patients (e.g. ethical issues, difficulties in recruitment and high attrition rates). It is important to remember that where drugs are used outside of their licensed indication, dose or route, then liability lies with the prescriber. An example of an off-licence indication would be amitriptyline for neuropathic pain. An example of an off-licence route would be midazolam by SC injection or infusion.

Use of medicines off-licence is both necessary and common in palliative care and pain management. Any healthcare professional involved in prescribing drugs beyond licence should select those drugs that offer the best balance of benefit against harm for any given patient.

## Prescribing issues from personal experience

### The patient

Identify as much of the patient's history as possible from all available sources to complete a comprehensive picture. Consultation with, and observation and examination of the patient are all important stages in the process. However, in very sick patients observation will be key, together with feedback from those caring for them.

### The patient's problems

Identification of all of the symptoms experienced is essential. Response to treatment must be assessed with regular review and monitoring for efficacy and tolerability of interventions. Attention to detail is a critical factor. Guidelines and evidence-based treatments, where available, should be followed, but treatment must be appropriate and individualised for the specific patient.

### The prescription

Ensure familiarity with drugs prescribed: pharmacodynamics, pharmaco-kinetics and pharmaceutical. Prescribe within your competence and refer on if unable to deal with the situation. Until the legislation regarding prescription of controlled drugs by pharmacist prescribers is changed, clinical management plans will still be required for most palliative care patients. Obtaining consent from patients who are very sick or lack capacity is an issue. It is good practice to obtain consent from the next of kin in these situations.

Continuing professional development is an integral part of the prescribing process and encourages the extension of knowledge and competence.

## Conclusion

Improving the quality of life for patients with life-limiting illnesses is an important objective for the multidisciplinary palliative care team. Well-managed symptom control is a major contributing factor. Prescribing for this group of patients presents a challenge. A pharmacist prescriber with the added value of pharmacological and pharmaceutical knowledge and attention to detail is well placed to safely provide continuing care for these patients.

# Case studies

## Case study 1

MM, 60-year-old female homecare patient, with adenocarcinoma of the stomach and adrenal and liver metastases.

### Past medical history
Chronic obstructive pulmonary disease, depression, weight loss, smoker, high alcohol intake. Currently still smoking heavily and high alcohol intake. No known drug allergies.

### Regular medications
- Fentanyl patch 125 µg/hour every 3 days
- Paracetamol 1 g four times daily
- Metoclopramide 10 mg three times a day
- Dexamethasone 4 mg every morning
- Omeprazole 40 mg every morning
- Venlafaxine 75 mg every morning and 150 mg every night
- Senna 2 every night
- Movicol 1 twice a day
- Aminophylline SR (Phyllocontin) 450 mg twice a day
- Evorel Conti patch Tuesday and Saturday.

### Medications as required
- Morphine normal release tablets (Sevredol) 70–100 mg
- Levomepromazine 6.25 mg.

### Presenting problems
- Right flank and upper abdominal pain, which comes on suddenly and rapidly increases in intensity. Episodic in nature, occurs 2–3 times a day. Regular bowel motions.
- MM takes Sevredol 70 mg when the pain starts, but this takes around 30 minutes to start working, and then the pain gradually subsides. For severe pain episodes, she takes Sevredol 100 mg, which relieves the pain but makes her very sleepy for several hours.
- Anxiety related to the intensity of pain and concerns about having an adequate supply of breakthrough medication.
- Occasional nausea despite regular metoclopramide.

Although somewhat chaotic, she is managing her medicines; the regular solid doses are dispensed in a Nomad compliance aid.

### 1 How would you deal with this?
Aim to reduce anxiety around pain episodes with better management of them. Sevredol works but takes time and the 100 mg dose makes her very

drowsy. To continue to take Sevredol 70 mg, but to add buccal alfentanil 2 to 4 sprays at onset of pain.

Each spray of alfentanil contains 140 µg/0.14 mL and should be sprayed into the inside of the cheek. Buccal absorption of alfentanil is rapid; a response is seen within minutes. Alfentanil has a short duration of action (1–2 hours). Using the two agents together may help to achieve faster pain control while maintaining relief for several hours.

Ensure adequate supply of breakthrough analgesia. Advise to request new supply well in advance (e.g. when starting last box of Sevredol).

Consider addition of regular levomepromazine 6.25 mg every night to try to improve control of nausea.

### 2 What are the prescribing issues?
- Clinical management plan required as alfentanil spray is made under a special licence by Torbay Hospital Manufacturing department.
- Written instructions required for use of alfentanil spray.
- Medication record to aid compliance with regimen.
- GP reluctant to prescribe alfentanil spray because of its unlicensed status.
- Pharmacist to prescribe to maintain supply.
- Letter to GP to request larger quantities of Sevredol on each prescription and the addition of regular levomepromazine at night to the regimen.

### 3 What would you prescribe?
- Alfentanil buccal spray 2–4 sprays as required.
- Supply three 5 mg/5 mL sprays.

### 4 What are the benefits to the patient?
- Better control of pain episodes and consequent reduction in anxiety.
- Rapid access to medicine supply.

## Case study 2

SD, 43-year-old female day care patient, with advanced cervical cancer and an ileal conduit urinary diversion following bilateral hydronephrosis. Weight 60.3 kg.

### Past medical history
- Depression, anxiety and panic attacks
- Bulimia, self-harm and neglect
- Mental health admission.

### Current medication (regular)
- Paracetamol 1 g four times daily
- Mirtazapine 30 mg every night

- Movicol 1–2 once daily (produces feeling of bloating)
- Metronidazole 400 mg three times daily (recently finished course)
- Senna 1–2 once daily.

**Current medication (as required)**
- Morphine normal release liquid (Oramorph) 5 mg
- Zopiclone 3.75 mg at night.

**Presenting problems**
- Vaginal pain described as tightness (like wearing tight underwear) and an ache with stabbing pains darting about. Pain radiating from groin to inside the vagina with a stabbing, tingling sensation.
- Malodorous vaginal discharge with red skin, nappy-like rash in the vaginal/groin area.
- Low mood, spends all day in bed, has no energy.
- Constipation.
- Poor compliance with medicine regimen.

**Clinical biochemistry**
- Sodium 136 (135–145) mmol/L
- Potassium 4.4 (3.5–5) mmol/L
- Urea 4.1 (2.5–6.6) mmol/L
- Creatinine 69 (60–120) μmol/L
- Alanine aminotransferase (ALT) 6 (<40) iu/L
- Bilirubin 4 (5–17) μmol/L
- Alkaline phosphatase 102 (30–130) iu/L
- Albumin 29 (35–51) g/L
- Corr. calcium 2.55 (2.15–2.55) mmol/L
- Phosphate 0.78 (0.8–1.40 mmol/L
- White blood count (WBC) 18.8 (5.1–11.4) $10^9$/L
- Haemoglobin 10.6 (11.5–15.1) g/dL
- Platelets 808 (147–397) $10^9$/L
- Neutrophils 17.0 (2.6–7.9) $10^9$/L
- Mean cell volume (MCV) 82 (84–98) fL
- C reactive protein (CRP) 140 (<10) mg/L.

**1 What can be done to improve her pain control?**
The patient has just started taking Oramorph 5 mg as required. It makes her drowsy and she feels tipsy. She describes the characteristics of neuropathic pain.

Encourage regular use of Oramorph every 4 hours and as required. Give reassurance about initial side-effects of opioids (i.e. drowsiness), which should resolve after a few days. Increase regular dose and as required according to severity and response. When opioid requirement determined, consider conversion to fentanyl patch, to aid compliance.

Consider addition of adjuvant agent for neuropathic pain. First-line options are amitriptyline or gabapentin. Amitriptyline is inappropriate as another antidepressant, mirtazapine, is already prescribed. There is increased risk of CNS sensitivity if used concomitantly.

For conservative gabapentin titration, to facilitate greater tolerability, commence with 100 mg at night for three nights, then 100 mg twice daily for 3 days, then 100 mg three times daily and review response.

Calculate creatinine clearance (CrCl) using Cockcroft–Gault equation to determine optimum dose range of gabapentin. CrCl calculated as 87 mL/min. Dose range of gabapentin 900–3600 mg for CrCl ≥80 mL/min. To increase dose within this range according to response and tolerability.

**2 What monitoring is required?**
The following variables will need to be monitored:
- pain score
- response to opioid
- as required requirements
- opioid adverse effects
- response to initiation of gabapentin
- renal function, in case of change; handling of morphine and gabapentin will be affected if renal function deteriorates
- gabapentin adverse effects.

**3 How should her constipation be managed and monitored?**
- For constipation: assess, review, titrate.
- Review Movicol as causes bloating. Stop senna and Movicol, consider co-danthramer, an agent that combines softener and stimulant, which will aid compliance.
- Monitor frequency and consistency of bowel motions.

**4 The vaginal discharge is embarrassing for her, what are the options?**
- Restart metronidazole orally or consider metronidazole gel intravaginally.
- Barrier cream for sore groin area: Siopel, lidocaine 2% in Lutrol gel (local anaesthetic in thermoplastic gel made by Guy's manufacturing department).

**5 What about her mood?**
The patient's mood may improve once better pain control achieved. There is also scope to increase mirtazapine up to 45 mg if necessary.

**6 What are the prescribing issues?**
- Multiple symptoms affecting quality of life.
- Clinical management plan required as controlled drugs to be prescribed.

- Appropriate dose of gabapentin for renal function.
- Close monitoring required to determine response to treatment and consequent increase in opioid and gabapentin doses.

### 7 What would you prescribe?

- Morphine normal release liquid (Oramorph) 5 mg every 4 hours + as required. Supply 300 mL (THREE HUNDRED MILLILITRES) of 10 mg/5 mL liquid.
- Gabapentin 100 mg every night for 3 days, then 100 mg twice daily for 3 days, then 100 mg three times daily.
- Co-danthramer 1–2 once daily.
- Metronidazole vaginal gel 0.75% every night.
- To continue with: paracetamol 1 g four times daily and mirtazapine 30 mg every night.

## Case study 3

SP, 83-year-old male resident in local nursing home with advanced vascular dementia.

### Past medical history

Parkinson's disease, cerebrovascular accidents (CVAs), type 2 diabetes mellitus and recurrent urinary tract infections (UTIs). Penicillin allergy.

### Current medication (regular)

- Aspirin 75 mg once daily
- Isosorbide mononitrate 60 mg once daily
- Atorvastatin 10 mg once daily
- Sodium valproate MR 500 mg once daily.

### Current medication (as required)

- Paracetamol 1 g up to four times daily
- Diazepam 5 mg rectally.

### Presenting problems

Deteriorating condition, appears to be entering terminal phase. After 4 days without oral fluids, GP prescribed glucose 5% 1 L by SC infusion over 24 hours after discussion with concerned daughter. Sleeping soundly and unresponsive on examination.

### 1 How would you deal with this?

Medication review required as patient no longer able to take oral medication. Consider end of life care. Daughter concerned about lack of hydration and the risk of further sedation with medicines. Review required:

- Oral regular medicines stopped as no longer able to take them.

- Consider midazolam 2.5 mg SC as required up to 2-hourly in case of fits or distress.
- Consider paracetamol 1 g rectally as required up to four times daily in case of discomfort.
- Hydration continued following discussion with daughter, but with NaCl 0.9% and at slow rate; 1 L over 24 hours for 2 days only then for further review.

### 2 What are the prescribing issues?

Clinical management plan for symptom control and patient comfort as controlled drugs prescribed. Consent to prescribe obtained from daughter as patient unable to give consent. Asked consultant to speak to daughter about hydration issues.

### 3 What would you prescribe?

Prescription (hospital inpatient type):
- NaCl 0.9% 1 L by SC infusion over 24 hours for 2 days
- midazolam 2.5 mg SC as required 2-hourly
- paracetamol 1 g rectally as required up to four times daily.

### 4 What are the benefits to the patient?

Input from specialist palliative care team for end of life care. Appropriate medication for symptom relief prescribed. Supply of medicines arranged from hospital pharmacy.

### Case study 4

JG, 53-year-old female homecare patient, with adenocarcinoma of the lung and bone, adrenal and brain metastases.

### Current medication (regular)
- Fentanyl patch 62µg/h every 3 days
- Paracetamol 1 g four times daily
- Dexamethasone 16 mg once daily
- Carbamazepine 200 mg once daily
- Omeprazole 20 mg once daily
- Co-danthramer 1–2 once daily
- Cyclizine 50 mg three times daily.

### Current medication (as required)
- Oxycodone normal release 15 mg
- Levomepromazine 6.25 mg.

### Presenting problems

Deteriorating condition, now unable to swallow oral medication. Back and leg pain controlled. Previous fits controlled. Occasional nausea. No known drug allergies.

### 1 How would you deal with this?

Aim to maintain symptom control in view of deteriorating condition and inability to swallow oral medication. Consider end of life care. Clinical management plan required because controlled drugs will need to be prescribed.

Review of medication required:

• Pain controlled, therefore continue with fentanyl patch.

As now unable to swallow:

• add oxycodone 7.5 mg SC as required (SC dose 50% of oral dose)
• stop co-danthramer, omeprazole and paracetamol
• add paracetamol rectally four times daily as required
• convert dexamethasone oral to SC injection or continuous SC infusion (CSCI) (this is preferable due to the volume of the injection: 4 mg/mL = 4 mL for 16 mg dose, inappropriate for SC injection)
• stop carbamazepine, start midazolam 10 mg by CSCI/24 hours to maintain seizure control
• stop cyclizine and change to levomepromazine 6.25 mg by CSCI/24 hours in view of occasional nausea despite regular cyclizine.

Ensure appropriate as required medication is available:

• midazolam 2.5 mg SC to treat fits and reduce anxiety or distress
• diazepam 5 mg rectal/sublingual (off-licence route) to treat fits
• glycopyrronium 400 µg SC up to three times daily in case of rattly, noisy breathing.

### 2 What are the prescribing issues?

Clinical management plan required as controlled drugs to be prescribed. Consent to prescribe obtained from husband as patient unable to give consent. Access to medicines for end of life care.

### 3 What would you prescribe?

• Syringe driver 1: dexamethasone 16 mg by CSCI over 24 hours
• Syringe driver 2: midazolam 10 mg by CSCI over 24 hours. Supply 10 (TEN) ampoules of 10 mg/2 mL injection
• levomepromazine 6.25 mg by CSCI over 24 hours
• midazolam 2.5 mg SC as required

- levomepromazine 3.125 mg SC as required
- oxycodone 7.5 mg SC as required. Supply 10 (TEN) ampoules of 10 mg/mL injection
- glycopyrronium 400 μg SC as required up to three times daily
- diazepam 5 mg rectally or sublingually as required
- sodium chloride 0.9% 10 mL – to make up syringe driver.

**4 What are the benefits to the patient?**
Continuity of care within the palliative care team. Continuity of symptom control at the end of life by the introduction of CSCI via syringe driver and injectable as required medication. Dispensed in the hospital pharmacy to ensure rapid access to medicines.

## Further reading

Clinical Knowledge Summaries. http://cks.library.nhs.uk/clinical_knowledge/clinical_topics/by_clinical_specialty/palliative_care.
Dickman A, Schneider J and Varga J (2005). *The Syringe Driver Continuous Subcutaneous Infusions in Palliative Care*, 2nd edn. New York: Oxford University Press.
Regnard C and Hockley J (2004). *A Guide to Symptom Relief in Palliative Care*, 5th edn. Oxford: Radcliffe Publishing.
Watson M, Lucas C and Hoy A (2006). *Adult Palliative Care Guidance*, 2nd edn. Oxford: Oxford University Press.

## Websites

Cancer Research UK. Information resource centre. http://info.cancerresearchuk.org/cancerstats.
National Council for Palliative Care (2006). http://www.ncpc.org.uk/.

## References

Atkinson C, Kirkham S (1999). Unlicensed uses for medication in a palliative care unit. *Palliative Med* 13: 145–152.
Baines MJ (1997). Clinical review: ABC of palliative care; nausea, vomiting and intestinal obstruction. *BMJ* 315: 1148–1150.
Donnelly S, Walsh D (1995). The symptoms of advanced cancer. *Semin Oncol* 22: 67–72.
National Council for Palliative Care (2006). http://www.ncpc.org.uk/palliative_care.html
Solano JP, Gomes B and Higginson IJ (2006). A comparison of symptom prevalence in far advanced cancer, AIDS, heart disease, chronic obstructive pulmonary disease and renal disease. *J Pain Symptom Manage* 31: 58–69.
Todd J and Davies A (1999). Use of unlicensed medication in palliative medicine. *Palliative Med* 13: 466.
Twycross R and Wilcock A (2001). *Symptom Management in Advanced Cancer*. Oxford: Radcliffe Publishing, pp. 141–154.
Twycross R and Wilcock A (2007). *Palliative Care Formulary*, 3rd edn. Oxford: Radcliffe Publishing.
Vainio A, Auvenun A and members of the symptom prevalence group (1996). Prevalence of symptoms among patients with advanced cancer: an international collaborative study. *J Pain Symptom Manage* 12: 3–10.

Van den Beuken-van Everdingen MHJ, de Rijke JM, Kessels AG, Schouten HC, van Kleef M and Patijn J (2007). Prevalence of pain in patients with cancer: a systematic review of the past 40 years. *Ann Oncol* 18: 1437–1449.

World Health Organization (WHO) (2005). WHO definition of palliative care. http://www.who.int/cancer/palliative/definition/en/.

Zech D, Grond S, Lynch J, Hertel D and Lehmann KA (1995). Validation of WHO guidelines for cancer pain relief; a 10 year prospective study. *Pain* 63: 65–76.

# 8

# Prescribing in cardiology

*Helen Williams*

---

**Key learning points:**

- Overview of the disease state

- Key issues for prescribing in this clinical area

- Overview of knowledge and skills for safe and effective prescribing

- Clinical case studies to demonstrate issues in non-medical prescribing

- Cardiology covers a wide range of clinical conditions, but the three areas in which non-medical prescribers are most likely to engage are:

  - Hypertension

  - Ischaemic heart disease (IHD)

  - Heart failure.

---

## Hypertension

Hypertension is defined as a 'sustained blood pressure of greater than 140/90 mmHg'. Most patients with hypertension will be asymptomatic, although some patients with very elevated pressures may complain of headaches. Most cases are therefore picked up on routine blood pressure checks, and an initial high reading should be confirmed by repeated readings taken on two further separate occasions before a diagnosis is made.

Hypertension is generally categorised as 'essential' hypertension, which accounts for 95% of cases and for which no known cause can be identified, or 'secondary' hypertension which accounts for the remaining 5% of cases and where a cause can be found. Key risk factors for developing hypertension include increasing age, Black African or Caribbean background and, for early onset hypertension, male gender. Blood pressure control in patients with hypertension is important to protect against the development of target organ damage and other long-term complications (*Box 8.1*).

> **Box 8.1** *Target organ damage and complications of hypertension*
> - Stroke, transient ischaemic attack (TIA), dementia, carotid bruits
> - Left ventricular hypertrophy and/or left ventricular strain on ECG, heart failure
> - Myocardial infarction, angina, coronary artery bypass graft or angioplasty
> - Peripheral vascular disease
> - Fundal haemorrhages or exudates, papilloedema
> - Proteinuria
> - Renal impairment (raised serum creatinine or reduced estimated glomerular filtration rate).

Key interventions to address high blood pressure are lifestyle modification and drug therapies.

Patients with blood pressure above 140/90 mmHg but lower than 160/100 mmHg without additional risk factors (no cardiovascular disease, diabetes, renal disease or at <20% risk of developing cardiovascular disease over the next 10 years) should be managed by addressing lifestyle issues alone.

Lifestyle advice should be given as part of a full discussion with the patient to identify any specific issues and emphasise the relative contribution of each risk factor to the development of hypertension. Areas to cover in discussion are:

- diet, particularly reducing salt intake
- weight reduction
- increasing physical activity
- smoking cessation
- moderating alcohol intake.

It is important not to underestimate how difficult lifestyle change can be, and patients should be encouraged to set realistic goals. Patients are unlikely to stick to an aggressive regimen that requires them to address every area of their lifestyle in one go. It may be appropriate to focus on one or two key areas and progress to other issues, as the patient succeeds in these areas (*Table 8.1*).

## Prescribing in hypertension

Drug therapy should be initiated where blood pressure is consistently >160/100 mmHg or in patients with blood pressure >140/90 mmHg where additional risk factors are present, such as established cardiovascular

| Table 8.1 Impact of lifestyle change on systolic blood pressure ||
| Intervention | Effect on systolic blood pressure |
| --- | --- |
| Weight reduction | 5–10 mmHg/10 kg weight loss |
| Diet rich in fruit and veg, low in dairy, reduced saturated fat | 8–14 mmHg |
| Restricted dietary sodium | 2–8 mmHg |
| Physical activity | 4–9 mmHg |
| Alcohol moderation | 2–4 mmHg |
| From Williams *et al.* (2004). ||

disease, diabetes, chronic kidney disease, or the patient is at >20% risk of developing cardiovascular disease. Once drug therapy is initiated, the aim is to lower blood pressure to less than 140/90 mmHg, with more aggressive targets for patients with diabetes (aim for blood pressure <140/80 mmHg or <130/80 mmHg if evidence of kidney, eye or cerebrovascular disease) or chronic kidney disease (aim for blood pressure <130/80 mmHg).

Choice of drug in the treatment of hypertension should be determined by the patient's age, ethnicity and co-morbidities. In line with the National Institute for Health and Clinical Excellence (NICE) algorithm, younger (<55 years) non-black patients should be offered treatment with an angiotensin-converting enzyme (ACE) inhibitor in the first instance (or an angiotensin receptor blocker if first-line ACE inhibitor is not tolerated) (NICE, 2006a). Older or black patients should be initiated on a thiazide diuretic or a calcium channel blocker.

Once initiated, drug therapy should be continued for at least four weeks before the efficacy in blood pressure lowering is assessed. Patients should be counselled that on initiation they may experience dizziness or lightheaded-ness for the first day or two as the blood pressure falls. In addition, common adverse effects should be discussed. For example, the impact of thiazide diuretic therapy on lifestyle should be considered, the possibility of ankle swelling with calcium channel blockers should be raised. Prior to and following initiation of ACE inhibitor, angiotensin receptor blocker and thiazide it is important to order blood tests to check renal function, in particular serum urea and creatinine, and serum potassium levels. ACE inhibitors and angiotensin receptor blockers can increase potassium levels significantly, especially in the setting of reduced renal function, while thiazide diuretics can lead to hypokalaemia. ACE inhibitors and calcium channel blockers should be started at low doses and therefore the dose needs to be titrated if blood pressure remains uncontrolled. There is little dose response in terms of blood pressure control with thiazide diuretics, but evidence of more side-effects at higher doses.

If blood pressure remains high on optimal first-line therapy, it is important to check that the patient is adhering to the prescribed medication in the first instance. If concordance is confirmed, then second-line therapy should be considered in line with the NICE algorithm. Most people with hypertension require two or more drugs to control blood pressure adequately. NICE guidance recommends that if a patient was initiated first-line on an ACE inhibitor, then the next step is to add a thiazide diuretic or a calcium channel blocker; or if started on one of the latter agents, then an ACE inhibitor should be added. Again, appropriate monitoring and dose titration should be undertaken. If blood pressure remains uncontrolled after optimising the second agent, then consideration should be given to adding in the missing agent from the group (ACE inhibitor, thiazide or calcium channel blocker, depending which agents have been used at steps 1 and 2). Lifestyle factors should be revisited at each step in the treatment pathway.

After the first three drugs have been initiated and optimised, if blood pressure remains uncontrolled, the clinician can consider adding in other agents such as alpha-blockers, beta-blockers or spironolactone. However, this may also be an appropriate time to consider referral for specialist advice, depending on the competence of the prescriber. Specialist hypertension or vascular risk clinics will focus on identifying underlying reasons for resistance to drug therapy. Certain patients are appropriate for earlier referral for specialist advice, in particular patients with early onset hypertension, such as white patients with hypertension below the age of 40 years old, or black patients with high blood pressure below the age of 30 years old. Hypertension in pregnancy should be referred for specialist management by an obstetrician, due to the risk of pre-eclampsia.

In addition to managing blood pressure, patients with hypertension require full cardiovascular risk assessment using a validated risk assessment tool, such as the Joint British Societies Risk Prediction Charts at the back of the BNF (Joint British Societies, 2005). Patients with a risk of developing cardiovascular disease of more than 20% over the next 10 years should be considered for treatment with a statin and low-dose aspirin (once blood pressure has been controlled to below 150/90 mmHg).

## Ischaemic heart disease

The management of ischaemic heart disease encompasses two specific issues:

- control of angina symptoms and
- secondary prevention of cardiovascular disease.

Anginal chest pain occurs when the oxygen demand of the heart exceeds that of supply usually, although not exclusively, as a result of an atheromatous narrowing (stenosis) in one or more of the coronary arteries. Estimated prevalence rates for angina vary significantly from study to study, but a figure of 4% of all adults in the UK has been calculated, equating to over 2 million angina patients across the UK. Patients with angina are at an increased risk of cardiovascular events in the future; hence in addition to managing angina symptoms (*Box 8.2*), secondary prevention of cardiovascular events is essential.

> **Box 8.2** *Common features of stable angina*
> - Central chest pain
> - Pain radiating to the lower jaw or arms
> - Shortness of breath
> - Lack of exercise tolerance
> - Provoked by exercise, stress, extremes of temperature
> - Relieved by rest, nitrates.

### Anti-anginal therapies

The symptoms of stable angina result from an imbalance between the oxygen requirements of the heart muscle and the supply it receives. Treatments are aimed at improving myocardial oxygen supply and/or reducing cardiac workload, hence lowering myocardial oxygen demand.

Acute chest pain should be treated initially with sublingual nitrate therapy, followed by chronic background therapy using beta-blockers, nitrates, calcium channel blockers, nicorandil and/or ivabradine to prevent recurrent episodes, except in those with very minimal and predictable symptoms manageable with sublingual nitrates alone.

There are few outcome data to guide choice of drug class to protect the patient against angina episodes, although most clinicians endorse the use of beta-blockers first-line where possible. This is based on extrapolation of outcomes achieved in post-myocardial infarction patients and the theoretical benefits of heart rate control in the setting of ischaemic heart disease. Choice of beta-blocker should take into account side-effect profile and ease of dosing, but key to protecting patients from ischaemic episodes is dose titration to achieve a resting heart of between 50 and 60 beats per minute. Common adverse effects include bradycardia and hypotension, cold extremities, lethargy/fatigue and impotence. Patients should be counselled to avoid abrupt cessation of beta-blocker therapy which has been associated with increased risk of cardiovascular events.

Where beta-blockers cannot be used due to contraindications or failure to tolerate therapy, rate-controlling calcium channel blockers, such as diltiazem or verapamil should be considered, or the more recently licensed ivabradine, a pure heart rate-lowering agent. If chest pain persists despite optimal first-line therapy, other agents can be added such as dihydropyridine calcium channel blockers (i.e. amlodipine), nitrates or nicorandil. In patients with recurrent episodes of angina, clinicians should have a low threshold for considering referral to a specialist for assessment of suitability for revascularisation (percutaneous coronary intervention or coronary artery bypass graft surgery).

## Secondary prevention strategies

Secondary prevention is defined as the prevention of the progression of a disease in symptomatic patients. In terms of ischaemic heart disease this applies to people who have survived a myocardial infarction and those who present with angina, have had a revascularisation by angioplasty and intra-coronary stent insertion or coronary artery bypass graft surgery, or patients with any other manifestation of atherosclerotic disease such as stroke, peripheral vascular disease or diabetes.

There are two aspects of secondary prevention: lifestyle changes and drug treatment. Examples of lifestyle changes to reduce cardiovascular risk include stopping smoking, increasing exercise, losing weight (if obese or overweight), improving diet (e.g. reducing total and saturated fat intake; increasing fruit, vegetable and fibre intake) and moderating alcohol consumption.

## Prescribing for secondary prevention

Unless there are contraindications, all patients with ischaemic heart disease should be prescribed a combination of secondary prevention drugs, which will include an antiplatelet agent, usually aspirin, a beta-blocker, a statin and an ACE inhibitor.

- Low-dose aspirin is the first-line antiplatelet agent in the majority of patients because it is effective, generally safe and inexpensive. A dose of 75 mg daily is recommended because it is proven to be equally effective as higher doses and is associated with a lower incidence of side-effects. Patients should be reminded to dissolve soluble aspirin and take it with or after food. Clopidogrel should only be used as an alternative to aspirin where there is evidence of true aspirin allergy.
- Beta-blockers are supported by strong evidence that they reduce the risk of overall mortality, coronary mortality, recurrent non-fatal myocardial infarction and sudden cardiac death in patients post-myocardial

infarction. Beta-blockers have a number of beneficial features including rate control (which may protect against ischaemic events), anti-arrhythmic properties and blood-pressure lowering. Beta-blockers should therefore be given to all patients following myocardial infarction, unless there are contraindications (e.g. uncontrolled heart failure). The benefits of beta-blockers post-myocardial infarction are also extrapolated to those patients with established ischaemic heart disease, and therefore beta-blockers are the first choice anti-anginal in patients with ischaemic symptoms.

- Statins are the only lipid-lowering class with consistent clinical trial data demonstrating a significant reduction in major cardiovascular outcomes, including reduced overall mortality, cardiovascular mortality and non-fatal cardiovascular events. All patients with coronary heart disease should have a full lipid profile performed, receive dietary advice and, if their total cholesterol or low-density lipoprotein (LDL) cholesterol is raised, should be prescribed a statin. Recent NICE guidance has recommended that all patients should be initiated on at least simvastatin 40 mg daily, although those post-acute coronary syndrome should be considered for higher intensity statin treatment such as atorvastatin 80 mg daily or an alternative agent which lowers cholesterol more than simvastatin 40 mg daily (for example, rosuvastatin 20 mg daily). Patients initiated on statin therapy for secondary prevention of cardiovascular disease should be treated with a view to achieving cholesterol targets of total cholesterol <4 mmol/L and LDL cholesterol <2 mmol/L to gain the greatest protection from cardiovascular events.

- ACE inhibitors were initially shown to protect against recurrent cardiovascular events and reduce mortality post-myocardial infarction. However, there is now substantial evidence that they protect patients with any manifestation of cardiovascular disease, except those where risk factors are aggressively controlled (i.e. blood pressure, cholesterol, blood sugar, etc.). Therefore, except where there is a contraindication, ACE inhibitors should be considered for all post-myocardial infarction patients, with or without symptoms of congestive heart failure or known left ventricular disease and all patients with established coronary heart disease.

## Heart failure

Despite major advances in the prevention and treatment of cardiac disease, the incidence and prevalence of heart failure continue to rise. Heart failure is associated with a high mortality rate – figures of up to 50% per annum are quoted. It is also responsible for frequent hospital admission and readmission and poor quality of life. Heart failure is characterised by breathlessness and reduced exercise tolerance, with the main sign being fluid retention, presenting as pulmonary or peripheral oedema.

Drug therapies in heart failure are targeted against two key pathways in disease progression:

- over-activity of the renin–angiotensin–aldosterone system (RAAS), which primarily causes vasoconstriction and sodium and water retention, further overloading the failing heart and
- increased sympathetic activation, which in turn increases blood pressure and heart rate and leads to further decline in left ventricular systolic function over time.

Symptom control in heart failure is achieved through the use of diuretics, mainly loop diuretics which are cheap, easy to use and relatively potent. Diuretic doses are titrated up and down to achieve an appropriate diuresis, sufficient to control heart failure symptoms without causing dehydration. Renal monitoring can be used to guide dosing. Diuretics have little, if any, effect on disease progression and therefore are not suitable for monotherapy in heart failure. All patients must also be started on other agents to improve longer term prognosis.

## Prescribing in heart failure

Two drug classes are the cornerstone of chronic heart failure management: ACE inhibitors and beta-blockers. In addition to these agents, spironolactone has a specific use for patients with severe heart failure.

### Angiotensin-converting enzyme inhibitors

Large-scale trials of ACE inhibitors in heart failure have demonstrated reductions in mortality, delayed disease progression, improvements in functional class and reduced hospitalisations in ACE-inhibitor-treated patients. These benefits are evident in all grades of heart failure (even asymptomatic heart failure) and have been shown for a number of different agents. ACE inhibitors should be started at a low dose with careful monitoring of blood pressure and renal function. Hypotension should not be considered a contraindication to therapy in this group of patients; ACE inhibitors can successfully be initiated in patients with systolic blood pressures as low as 90 mmHg. The specific diagnosis of bilateral renal artery stenosis is a contraindication to ACE inhibitor therapy, but renal dysfunction in itself is not, although in more severe cases (serum creatinine >250 mmol/L) specialist advice should be sought. Once initiated, ACE inhibitor therapy should be continued indefinitely.

ACE inhibitors should be titrated to achieve the maximum tolerated dose within the licensed dose range; higher doses have been shown to reduce hospital admission rates, when compared with lower doses. The key adverse effect which impacts on patient concordance is the development of an ACE-inhibitor-induced cough. Patients should be advised to persist with ACE inhibitor therapy where possible, but if the cough is troublesome an angiotensin receptor blocker (ARB) can be considered as an alternative. Currently only candesartan and losartan are licensed for this indication. Under specialist supervision, there is also evidence that ACE inhibitor and ARB combination therapy can further improve outcomes over ACE inhibitor therapy alone, although in this circumstance hypotension, renal dysfunction and hyperkalaemia become more problematic.

### Beta-blockers

Beta-blockers were established as key to heart failure management in the late 1990s when studies demonstrated significant reductions in mortality, reduced hospitalisations and improved symptom control. The benefits of beta-blocker therapy have been established in all functional classes of heart failure, except asymptomatic disease and are evident in a wide range of patient populations including diabetics, the elderly and those with renal dysfunction. Beta-blockers should therefore be considered for all patients with symptomatic heart failure. Ideally, these agents should be initiated when patients are clinically stable and optimised on first-line therapy (primarily ACE inhibitors and diuretics). Data exist to support the use of bisoprolol, carvedilol, metoprolol and more recently in the elderly population, nebivolol, however metoprolol remains unlicensed for this indication in the UK.

Beta-blocker therapy should be initiated at low doses and titrated slowly over approximately three months to achieve a resting heart rate between 50–60 beats per minute. Low starting doses are necessary to prevent precipitation of an acute episode of heart failure. Due to the effect of beta-blockers on heart rate and force of contraction, patients may experience an exacerbation of symptoms during the dose titration phase. Additional diuretic therapy may aid in the resolution of such symptoms. Beta-blockers are considered to be contraindicated in patients with severe bradycardia, acute heart failure, severe asthma or bronchospasm and peripheral vascular disease. Mild to moderate airways disease is not a contraindication, but prescribers should consider prescribing a cardioselective agent, such as bisoprolol, with careful monitoring of respiratory function.

### Spironolactone

Spironolactone, an aldosterone antagonist, has been shown to confer a mortality benefit when prescribed to patients with moderate to severe heart failure (in addition to ACE inhibitor and beta-blocker). In addition spironolactone-treated patients had fewer hospital admissions for cardiac events. Low-dose spironolactone should be considered for addition to optimised ACE inhibitor therapy in patients with moderate to severe heart failure symptoms following an acute hospitalisation. For this indication, spironolactone should be prescribed at an initial dose of 25 mg daily, titrated to 50 mg daily if symptoms persist after a number of weeks of therapy. Renal function and serum potassium should be monitored carefully throughout therapy. Should hyperkalaemia (serum potassium >5.5 mmol/L) occur, a dosage reduction to 25 mg on alternative days should be considered. Declining renal function, hyperkalaemia and the occurrence of painful gynaecomastia frequently result in withdrawal of spironolactone therapy in clinical practice. Spironolactone is contraindicated in hyperkalaemia, hyponatraemia and Addison's disease.

## Other issues

In addition to managing the clinical syndrome of heart failure, it is essential to identify and where possible treat the underlying cause. Common causes of chronic heart failure in the UK are ischaemic heart disease and hypertension (see previous sections), but other causes include excessive alcohol intake, viral infection and valvular heart disease. All patients should be reviewed by a specialist early following diagnosis to assess whether other therapeutic strategies are warranted such as revascularisation for ischaemic patients or the use of implantable devices to manage symptoms. Due to the poor prognosis for heart failure patients, palliative issues should also be considered throughout treatment.

## Case studies

### Case study 1

Patient RB is a 46-year-old African man who has had two high blood pressure readings recorded within the GP surgery in the past and has been given appropriate lifestyle advice. He is attending on this occasion for a further blood pressure check to confirm a diagnosis of hypertension. The patient is currently asymptomatic – his high blood pressure was picked up in the gym where he was offered a blood pressure check when he enrolled.

### On examination
His blood pressure readings recorded at this visit were:

- initial 180/100 mmHg
- second 168/96 mmHg

- third 166/102 mmHg
- BMI: 32kg/m$^2$
- abdominal circumference: 107 cm.

His mother died of a stroke at the age of 52 in Ghana. He is a non-smoker. His bloods were ordered following his previous clinic visit, a month ago.

**Biochemistry**
- Sodium 136 mmol/L
- Potassium 4.6 mmol/L
- Urea 4.2 mmol/L
- Serum creatinine 112 μmol/L
- Estimated glomerular filtration rate (eGFR) 58 mL/min (unadjusted)
- Total cholesterol 5.6 mmol/L
- High-density lipoprotein (HDL) 0.9 mmol/L
- Low-density lipoprotein (LDL) 3.2 mmol/L
- Triglycerides 2.1 mmol/L
- Liver function tests: NAD (nothing abnormal detected)
- Thyroid function tests: NAD (nothing abnormal detected)
- Fasting glucose 4.9 mmol/L.

On discussion, the patient reports being a non-smoker and an occasional drinker (2–4 units per week). He is a bus driver by occupation.

**1 What is the diagnosis?**
The diagnosis of hypertension is now clear, as high blood pressure readings have been documented on three separate occasions.

**2 What information should be given to this patient about the implications of the diagnosis?**
It is important to discuss the implications of such a diagnosis with the patient, in particular, highlighting the increased risk of stroke and heart attack, plus the potential damage to the kidneys if this is left untreated. This is an asymptomatic condition and without understanding the long-term adverse effects of high blood pressure, there is little incentive for a patient to make the necessary lifestyle changes to reduce their risk, or comply with any drug therapies prescribed.

Lifestyle factors are important in the management of hypertension and these should be identified and appropriate advice given.

**3 What are the prescribing issues?**
As this patient had a blood pressure >160/100 mmHg, he met the criteria for initiation of drug therapy. Drug choice should take into account the patient's age and ethnicity, alongside other issues such as co-morbidities. According to NICE guidelines, in a Black African patient first-line treatment

should be a thiazide diuretic, such as bendroflumethiazide, or a calcium channel blocker, such as amlodipine.

However, a thiazide diuretic might be inappropriate here, as the patient is a bus driver and frequent trips to the toilet would be difficult to manage. For this reason the decision was taken to initiate amlodipine at a dose of 5 mg daily. Care was taken when prescribing to ensure the generic amlodipine preparation would be dispensed. The patient was advised that the drug may cause some adverse effects in the first few days, in particular dizziness or lightheadedness as the blood pressure reduced, headaches and flushing. He was advised that these are usually short-lived. In the longer term, the most frequently cited side-effect is ankle swelling and if this occurred and was troublesome, he was advised to seek further advice.

The patient was booked in for a review in one month's time. Bearing in mind his pre-treatment blood pressure, the use of amlodipine at this dose is unlikely to achieve target blood pressure. Most patients require two or more antihypertensives to achieve the blood pressure treatment target of <140/90 mmHg. No specific biochemical monitoring is required following amlodipine initiation, so no blood tests were ordered at this stage.

At the next clinic visit, it will be important to review his blood pressure control, discuss his progress with lifestyle issues, assess the effectiveness and tolerability of the prescribed drug therapy and consider his global cardiovascular risk by undertaking a cardiovascular risk assessment.

## Case study 2

Mr AR, a 62-year-old white British man with known hypertension (pretreatment level 170/88 mmHg), was scheduled in for a review of his blood pressure management. He had been seen a number of times before, and had known concordance issues. At the last visit a month ago, his blood pressure was controlled to Quality and Outcomes framework target of 150/90 mmHg for the first time, but was not yet achieving the clinical target of 140/90 mmHg. At the last visit ramipril was added to his drug therapy. Low levels of physical activity. Non-smoker. Alcohol intake ~20 units per week.

### Current drug list
- Bendroflumethiazide 2.5 mg daily
- Amlodipine 5 mg daily
- Ramipril 2.5 mg daily.

### Bloods from two weeks ago
- Sodium 144 mmol/L
- Potassium 4.1 mmol/L (previously 3.7 mmol/L)
- Urea 5.3 mmol/L

- Serum creatinine 98 μmol/L (previously 93 μmol/L)
- eGFR 62 mL/min (previously 63 mL/min)
- Total cholesterol 5.4 mmol/L
- HDL 0.9 mmol/L
- LDL 3.2 mmol/L
- Triglycerides 2.1 mmol/L
- Liver function tests: NAD (nothing abnormal detected)
- Thyroid function tests: NAD (nothing abnormal detected)
- Fasting glucose 6.1 mmol/L
- BMI 36
- Abdominal girth 112 cm.

**On examination**
His blood pressure readings recorded at this visit were:

- initial 141/76 mmHg
- second 136/77 mmHg
- third 135/72 mmHg.

**1 How would you assess the patient's cardiovascular risk?**
The patient's blood pressure is now well controlled. However, this clinic visit is important in terms of allowing a full assessment of his cardiovascular risk. He has a number of risk factors including male gender, age, known hypertension, adverse lipid profile (raised total cholesterol, LDL and triglycerides and low levels of protective LDL), obesity and raised abdominal girth and low levels of physical activity. The patient's cardiovascular risk should be calculated using a validated risk assessment tool, such as the cardiovascular risk prediction charts issued by the Joint British Societies, which can be found at the back of the BNF. Risk assessment should be performed using untreated blood pressure and lipid levels.

**2 What are the implications of this patient's cardiovascular risk?**
For this patient, the Joint British Societies risk prediction charts indicate a cardiovascular risk of over 30% over the next 10 years, using pretreatment levels. Patients with cardiovascular risk greater than 20% should be considered high risk and be offered primary prevention. In this case, this would mean initiation of low-dose aspirin and a statin. Aspirin should only be started for primary prevention in hypertensive patients when the blood pressure has been lowered to below 150/90 mmHg to reduce the risk of intracranial haemorrhage. Statin therapy should be started, in line with NICE TA94, using a 'low acquisition cost statin' such as simvastatin (NICE, 2006b).

**3 What is the prescribing issue?**
The patient is known to have a history of poor compliance with drug therapy. It is therefore important to clearly explain his high risk of developing

cardiovascular disease over the next 10 years, and the benefits afforded by treatment with aspirin and a statin. Care should be taken to advise the patient on potential adverse effects and how to deal with them.

Aspirin should be taken with or after food to reduce the risk of gastrointestinal discomfort. Simvastatin should ideally be taken with the evening meal, but in this case, to aid compliance the patient was advised to take the simvastatin in the morning with all his other medications. For simvastatin, the evidence suggests that a dose taken in the evening lowers cholesterol marginally more than the same dose taken in the morning. This effect may be clinically significant – one study showed a difference in total cholesterol of 0.38 mmol/L and LDL cholesterol of 0.25 mmol/L when comparing morning and evening efficacy. Morning dosing should be considered in patients with compliance problems – better to have a (large) partial effect, than no effect at all because the patient always forgets their evening dose. The patient was also advised to seek medical advice should muscle pain or aches occur.

### 4 What monitoring and follow-up should there be?

Care was also taken to arrange appropriate monitoring and follow-up. Liver function should be checked at baseline and after one month of therapy, to ensure no adverse effect. The patient should be reviewed in 4–6 weeks to reinforce the need for therapy, check compliance and assess tolerability. Finally, lifestyle advice should not be forgotten; issues for this patient are weight loss and physical activity.

### Case study 3

Mrs PH, a 62-year-old white woman, attends your clinic for review and re-supply of drug therapy having been discharged from hospital following an acute myocardial infarction (MI) three weeks previously. The scanned discharge summary confirms ST-elevation MI, which was treated by primary angioplasty and bare metal stent insertion. She had an uncomplicated recovery and was discharged on the following drug therapy.

### Current drug list
* Aspirin 300 mg daily for one month then 75 mg daily thereafter
* Clopidogrel 75 mg daily for one month then stop
* Ramipril 2.5 mg daily
* Bisoprolol 2.5 mg daily
* Simvastatin 40 mg daily
* Fluoxetine 20 mg daily
* Omeprazole 20 mg daily.

Only fluoxetine and omeprazole were prescribed prior to this hospital admission. Blood pressure today: 110/68 mmHg; heart rate: 67 beats per minute.

The length of hospital stay following an acute MI has reduced significantly in centres performing primary angioplasty – often patients are discharged on day 2 or 3. This leaves very little time to optimise drug therapy and this issue now needs to be addressed in primary care.

**1 How should this patient's drug therapy be reviewed?**
This patient's drug therapy needs to be reviewed and some agents should be dose titrated to ensure she gets the maximum protection from future cardiovascular events.

As the patient was discharged over three weeks ago, her aspirin dose should soon be reduced to 75 mg daily and clopidogrel therapy should be stopped in a week's time. Most hospitals supply the full duration of clopidogrel therapy, when only one month's treatment is required, so no further prescriptions should be necessary in primary care. Ramipril should be dose titrated over the next few weeks to achieve a target dose of 10 mg daily. However, the dose should not be changed until the patient's renal function has been checked, to ensure no adverse effect since the ACE inhibitor was started in hospital. This will have to be dealt with at a future visit. The bisoprolol dose should similarly be dose titrated, aiming for a target heart rate of 55–60 beats per minute. This could be undertaken today after a check of blood pressure and heart rate. Dose titration can be undertaken provided systolic blood pressure is >90 mmHg and pulse rate is >60 beats per minute.

The efficacy of simvastatin therapy cannot be assessed at this stage as lipid levels fall naturally for a few weeks post-MI. The lipid levels should be re-checked at least three months after the MI, and dose titration of simvastatin, or use of an alternative agent considered at that point. However, liver function can be checked at this point to ensure no adverse effects.

**2 What assessments should be made during the consultation?**
In the consultation it was important to assess how the patient had been coping since discharge, both physically and psychologically. The patient was encouraged to attend a cardiac rehabilitation programme to assist with this. In terms of drug therapy, compliance with the new drug therapy regimen was assessed and appeared to be good. The patient was also encouraged to discuss any concerns or adverse effects but had no issues to raise. The importance of secondary prevention to protect against future events was emphasised, and the need for dose titration explained.

The following blood tests were ordered: full blood count and a biochemistry profile (including renal and liver function). A prescription for aspirin 75 mg daily, ramipril 2.5 mg daily, bisoprolol 5 mg daily (dose increased) and simvastatin 40 mg daily was issued, alongside other repeat medications. The patient was counselled that blood pressure may fall following the increase in beta-blocker dose, and as a result she may feel a little dizzy or lightheaded. Other side-effects discussed were increased tiredness and lethargy, and cold fingers and toes. A further clinic appointment was booked in four weeks with a view to increasing the ramipril dose.

## Case study 4

Mr JT, a 52-year-old white man, a builder, was diagnosed with hypertension for many years and more recently developed angina, diagnosed following an exercise tolerance test in a rapid access chest pain clinic. Following diagnosis, the clinic started him on atenolol 50 mg daily, aspirin 75 mg daily, simvastatin 40 mg daily and glyceryl trinitrate (GTN) spray when required to treat acute chest pain. Since it was first identified, his hypertension has been mild at approximately 150/95 mmHg and has therefore not previously warranted drug therapy. He was reviewed in clinic to assess his response to the new agents introduced recently and ensure all his cardiovascular risk factors are being fully addressed.

### On examination
His blood pressure was 146/84 mmHg; heart rate 75 bpm; BMI 28; and abdominal girth 86 cm.

The patient reported partial resolution of his angina symptoms, which were entirely exertion related. He was now only experiencing chest pain once or twice a week, compared with almost daily prior to starting atenolol. He had been feeling a little lethargic over the past few weeks, but thought this had improved over time. On discussion it transpires that he is still smoking, although he does express a desire to quit. He has never received any formal smoking cessation advice or nicotine replacement therapy. Also, he has a high alcohol intake of approximately 40 units per week.

### 1 What are the key issues?
Key issues here were:

- lifestyle issues, in particular smoking and alcohol intake
- blood pressure control – as this patient now has established cardiovascular disease, the threshold for initiating drug therapy falls from 160/100 mmHg to 140/90 mmHg
- optimising anti-anginal therapy to further reduce chest pain frequency
- ensuring secondary prevention strategies are optimised and encourage compliance.

### 2 What are the treatment options?
The patient was started on atenolol for the treatment of his angina, which had some impact on his blood pressure; but still did not achieve target blood pressure levels. The options now are to increase the atenolol to deal with any residual angina, or initiate another antihypertensive agent. Atenolol dose titration above 50 mg daily has little additional impact on blood pressure

control. Also, the patient had been concerned regarding tiredness since the atenolol was started, which was affecting his work as a builder. In this case, therefore, it seemed appropriate to consider an additional agent. While bendroflumethiazide may be the most cost-effective option here, the combination of beta-blocker and thiazide is known to increase the risk of diabetes. In addition, the use of amlodipine will assist in treating the angina symptoms, as well as the blood pressure. On discussion with the patient, it was decided to add amlodipine 5 mg daily. The patient was warned about the possibility of ankle swelling, headache and flushing with the new treatment.

In terms of secondary prevention, he is already treated with aspirin and a statin. The introduction of an ACE inhibitor for further cardiovascular risk reduction may be warranted in future. He needed blood tests ordering. As he had been newly started on simvastatin and had a history of excess alcohol intake, liver function tests were ordered, alongside a routine full blood count and biochemistry. The patient expressed understanding of his drug therapy and a willingness to comply.

### 3 What are the counselling points?

It was suggested that he consider seeing the smoking cessation adviser for the practice, with view to the use of nicotine replacement or drug therapy such as varenicline to improve his chance of quitting smoking. Alcohol moderation was advised to within the currently recommended limits of 21 units per week for a male. These issues should be followed up in one month, when the next blood pressure check is due.

## Case study 5

Mr DS, a 72-year-old white man with alcoholic heart failure and ischaemic heart disease, was listed for review in clinic. He was diagnosed with heart failure on echocardiogram 3 years ago (ejection fraction 28%).

### Current drug list
- Ramipril 5 mg daily (reduced from 5 mg twice daily two months ago)
- Nebivolol 10 mg once daily
- Furosemide 80 mg daily
- Spironolactone 12.5 mg daily (reduced from 25 mg daily four weeks ago)
- Aspirin 75 mg daily
- Simvastatin 20 mg daily
- Salbutamol inhaler 1 or 2 puffs four times daily
- Seretide 250 inhaler 1 puff twice daily
- Omeprazole 20 mg daily
- Senna 1 or 2 tablets at night as required.

His symptoms have been well controlled for the past six months, since his last admission to hospital with decompensated heart failure.

At this visit, Mr DS is asymptomatic, able to walk for over 20 minutes on the flat without symptoms of breathlessness or chest pain; and climb a flight of stairs without stopping. He reports that he is still drinking an average of 3 pints of draft lager each day. His blood pressure is well controlled at 110/68 mmHg sitting, but there is a significant postural drop, with a blood pressure of 96/54 mmHg on standing associated with dizziness/lightheadedness.

### Bloods from a week ago

- Sodium 129 mmol/L (down) (previously in normal range)
- Potassium 5.4 mmol/L (up) (reduced from 5.6 mmol/L one month ago)
- Urea: 12.9 mmol/L (up) (reduced from 14.1 mmol/L one month ago)
- Serum creatinine 197 micromol/L (up) (increased from 164 mmol/L one month ago)
- eGFR: 28 mL/min (down) (reduced from 36 mL/min one month ago)
- Liver function tests: bilirubin 5 μmol/L
- Albumin 38 g/L (down)
- Alanine aminotransferase (ALT) 8 iu/L
- Alkaline phosphatase 80 iu/L
- Gamma-glutamyl transferase (GGT) 136 iu/L (up)
- Thyroid function tests: NAD (nothing abnormal detected).

Lipids were controlled on current statin therapy.

### 1 What do the blood test results suggest?

The bloods demonstrate a deterioration in renal function, with raised serum creatinine and urea, hyperkalaemia and hyponatraemia with a significantly reduced eGFR. This, together with the postural blood pressure drop, suggests that the patient is dehydrated. The case highlights the difficult balance between optimal heart failure management to improve prognosis and quality of life (ACE inhibitor, spironolactone, diuretic therapy) and the risk of adverse drug effects if the doses are pushed too high.

### 2 What are the key issues?

Key issues to address here are:

- balancing diuretic use to control symptoms but avoid dehydration
- management of hyponatraemia and hyperkalaemia
- protection of renal function in view of evidence of increased serum urea and creatinine
- counselling on the risks of continuing to drink in the setting of alcoholic heart failure.

3 What are the drug treatment review options?

In this case, the most important therapies to maintain at optimal doses are the ACE inhibitor and beta-blocker as these are known to improve symptom control and prolong life. Reducing the furosemide dose in the first instance would seem a logical step forward, as the patient appears to be dehydrated. This will also assist in correcting the hyponatraemia, but may further exacerbate the hyperkalaemia as the diuresis falls. Spironolactone in the setting of dehydration will contribute to the hyponatraemia and hyperkalaemia and may also adversely affect the renal function. Whether to withdraw the spironolactone at this point depends on a balance of risks. As the patient is relatively stable from a heart failure point of view, it may be considered safer to withdraw the spironolactone therapy in the short term to reduce the pressure on the kidneys and minimise the risk of hyperkalaemia. Careful follow-up is important here to ensure renal function improves, no worsening of hyperkaleamia and, of course, to ensure that heart failure symptoms do not worsen.

In the clinic, the patient's furosemide was reduced to 40 mg daily and the spironolactone withdrawn. Repeat blood tests were ordered for 10 days' time and review in clinic booked for two weeks time with a view to reintroducing the spironolactone for its prognostic benefits if renal function has improved and sodium and potassium levels have normalised. The patient was advised to reduce, or ideally stop, his alcohol intake, and reminded to keep active.

This is a complex case with a high risk of destabilising heart failure control or precipitating renal failure. Non-medical prescribers should consider whether the management of this patient is within their scope of practice, or whether further advice should be sought from the GP or specialist heart failure service.

## Further reading

### Hypertension

British Hypertension Society Guidelines Working Party (2004). Guidelines for management of hypertension: Report of the Fourth Working Party of the British Hypertension Society, 2004 – BHS IV. *J Human Hypertens* 18: 139–185.

National Institute for Health and Clinical Excellence (NICE) (2006). Clinical Guideline 34: Hypertension Management of Hypertension in Adults in Primary Care. London: National Institute for Health and Clinical Excellence.

NICE (2006). TA94: Cardiovascular Disease – Statins for the prevention of cardiovascular events in patients at increased risk of developing cardiovascular disease or those with established cardiovascular disease. London: National Institute for Health and Clinical Excellence.

NICE (2008). Clinical Guideline 66: Type 2 Diabetes. Management of Type 2 Diabetes. London: National Institute for Health and Clinical Excellence.

## Ischaemic heart disease

Department of Health (2000). National Service Framework for Coronary Heart Disease: Modern standards and service models. http://www.dh.gov.uk/en/Publicationsandstatistics/Publications/PublicationsPolicyAndGuidance/DH_4094275 (accessed 17 May 2007).

Joint British Societies (2005). JBS-2 guidelines on the prevention of cardiovascular disease in clinical practice. *Heart* 91: v1–53.

National Institute for Health and Clinical Excellence (NICE) (2006). TA94: Cardiovascular Disease – Statins for the prevention of cardiovascular events in patients at increased risk of developing cardiovascular disease or those with established cardiovascular disease. London: National Institute for Health and Clinical Excellence.

NICE (2007). Clinical Guideline 48: MI: secondary prevention in primary and secondary care for patients following a myocardial infarction. London: National Institute for Health and Clinical Excellence.

NICE (2008). Clinical Guideline 67: Lipid Modification: Cardiovascular risk assessment and the modification of blood lipids for the primary and secondary prevention of cardiovascular disease. London: National Institute for Health and Clinical Excellence.

## Heart failure

Department of Health (2000). National Service Framework for Coronary Heart Disease: Modern standards and service models. Chapter 6: Heart failure. http://www.dh.gov.uk/en/Publicationsandstatistics/Publications/PublicationsPolicyAndGuidance/DH_4094275 (accessed 17 May 2007).

European Society of Cardiology (2008). ESC guidelines for the diagnosis and treatment of acute and chronic heart failure 2008. *Eur Heart J* 29: 2388–2442.

NICE (2003). Clinical Guideline 5: Chronic Heart Failure: Management of chronic heart failure in adults in primary and secondary care. London: National Institute for Health and Clinical Excellence.

# References

Joint British Societies (2005). JBS-2 guidelines on the prevention of cardiovascular disease in clinical practice. *Heart* 91: v1–53.

National Institute for Health and Clinical Excellence (NICE) (2006a). Clinical Guideline 34: Hypertension Management of Hypertension in Adults in Primary Care. London: National Institute for Health and Clinical Excellence.

NICE (2006b). TA94: Cardiovascular Disease – Statins for the prevention of cardiovascular events in patients at increased risk of developing cardiovascular disease or those with established cardiovascular disease. London: National Institute for Health and Clinical Excellence.

Williams B, Poulter N R, Brown M J, Davis M, McInnes G T, Potter J P, Sever P S and Thom S McG (2004). The BHS Guidelines Working Party Guidelines for Management of Hypertension: Report of the Fourth Working Party of the British Hypertension Society, BHS IV. *J Human Hypertens* 18: 139–185.

# 9

# Respiratory disease management

*Nader Siabi*

---

**Key learning points:**

- Overview of the disease state

- Key issues for prescribing in this clinical area

- Overview of knowledge and skills for safe and effective prescribing

- Clinical case studies to demonstrate issues in non-medical prescribing.

---

## Introduction

Asthma and chronic obstructive pulmonary disease (COPD) are two distinct respiratory conditions that share a number of similar signs and symptoms. Although both conditions are treated with inhaled medications, because of the nature and the cause of each condition, the treatment strategies are slightly different. The following competencies are essential in delivering effective respiratory clinics:

- understanding of consultation processes and effective history taking
- understanding of spirometric testing and patient preparations
- interpretation of peak expiratory flow rate (PEFR) and spirometric results
- understanding of NICE, SIGN and BTS guidelines on asthma, allergic rhinitis and COPD
- respiratory diseases treatment pathways
- effective patient communications and production of individualised treatment plans.

# Is it asthma or COPD?

## Signs and symptoms

Asthma is a chronic inflammatory disease of the lung characterised by eosinophilic infiltration of the airway walls, and airway narrowing. The narrowing is caused by a combination of factors that include spasm of smooth muscles surrounding the airways, oedema of mucosal membrane, formation of mucus plaques and secretions and gradual injury and shedding of the airways epithelial wall. Because of the inflammatory nature of asthma, it is easily treatable with effective anti-inflammatory medications. One significant characteristic of asthma disease is hyperresponsiveness to asthma-triggering factors, if the inflammation is not treated effectively. These two factors – inflammatory episodes and bronchial hyperresponsiveness – lead to classic symptoms of asthma that include cough, expiratory wheeze, chest tightness and shortness of breath.

Where the condition is under-treated, persistent or poorly managed, it will lead to structural changes that are characterised by the thickening of basement membrane and hypertrophy of the airways smooth muscle, resulting in irreversible fibrosis not fully reversible with medication (Jeffery, 1998). Characteristics of asthma are that symptoms tend to be variable in nature, intermittent, appear to be worse at night (early morning awakening and shortness of breath) and are mainly provoked by triggers including exercise, pollutants, allergens and other environmental factors (SIGN and BTS, 2007).

COPD is an umbrella term used to describe collective diseases of airways including chronic bronchitis, emphysema and bronchiectasis, chronic obstructive airway disease and chronic airway flow limitation (British Thoracic Society, 1997). The working definition of COPD is a slowly progressive disorder characterized by airflow obstruction (reduced force expiratory volume in one second ($FEV_1$) and $FEV_1$/forced vital capacity (FVC) ratio) that does not vary markedly over several months of observation (British Thoracic Society, 1997). Airflow obstruction is defined as a reduced $FEV_1$ and a reduced $FEV_1$/FVC ratio, such that $FEV_1$ is less than 80% predicted and $FEV_1$/FVC is less than 0.7 (NICE, 2004). COPD is different to asthma in that in COPD cell walls are infiltrated mainly by neutrophils, whereas asthma is eosinophilic in nature. Unlike asthma, the airflow obstruction in COPD is irreversible (or slightly reversible) upon administration of bronchial dilator and signs and symptoms are progressive in nature that vary very little with time but progressively become worse. Like asthma, cough, wheeze and shortness of breath may present, but the large variability seen in asthma is not usually seen in COPD. Other symptoms include increased sputum production, dyspnoea, poor exercise tolerance and right-sided heart failure (NICE, 2004; SIGN and BTS, 2007). The clinical features used to

**Table 9.1** Clinical features differentiating COPD and asthma

|  | COPD | Asthma |
|---|---|---|
| Smoker or ex-smoker | Nearly all | Possibly |
| Symptoms under age 35 years | Rare | Often |
| Chronic productive cough | Common | Uncommon |
| Breathlessness | Persistent and progressive | Variable |
| Night-time waking with breathlessness and/or wheeze | Uncommon | Common |
| Significant diurnal or day-to-day variability of symptoms | Uncommon | Common |

From Bellamy *et al.*, 2005. Reproduced with permission from the British Thoracic Society.

differentiate COPD and asthma are listed in *Table 9.1*. Please note that some asthmatic patients with allergic rhinitis may exhibit persistent productive cough, this should not be confused with productive cough seen in COPD patients.

## Prevalence, cause, detection and prevention

Asthma is very common among patients with a family history of asthma or those with other atopic conditions (eczema, allergic rhinitis) (British Thoracic Society, 2008). In those with a family link of asthma, the risk of the second child suffering from frequent wheezing reduces with age, being high at the age of 2 and significantly lower from the age of 6 through to the age of 13 (Ball *et al.*, 2000). This suggests that exposure to other children in the family may protect against the development of asthma and frequent wheezing later in childhood, although bronchial hyperresponsiveness was unaffected among the children (Koppelman *et al.*, 2001).

COPD is mainly caused by continuous smoking; more than 90% of confirmed cases of COPD are either smokers or ex-smokers (British Thoracic Society, 1997; Anthonisen *et al.*, 2005; Wilts *et al.*, 2005). The remaining 10% have a genetic predisposition mainly caused by alpha-antitrypsin deficiency. The absolute risk of developing COPD amongst continuous smokers is estimated as being at least 25–41% (Lokke *et al.*, 2006), after 25 years of follow-up, far more than the previous estimate of 15% (British Thoracic Society, 1997).

Asthmatic smokers and ex-smokers are more resistant to steroid therapy than non-smokers. Furthermore, exposure of children to cigarette smoke (passive smoking) in the first 3 years of life is considered a risk factor for atopy irrespective of family size (Koppelman *et al.*, 2001) and if the mother smokes during the pregnancy this is a risk factor for the development of wheezing in the first year of a child's life (Dezateux *et al.*, 1999).

Diagnosis of asthma in adults and children over 5 years of age involves objective tests that include measurement of peak expiratory flow rate (PEFR) and $FEV_1$, combined with clinical features that are indicative of asthma. Where a spirometric test is available, it is preferred to peak flow measurement and provides better and more accurate objective data. This is mainly due to variability of PEFR data in individual patients with time and circumstances of testing. PEFR is the preferred method for patient follow-ups to evaluate effectiveness of treatment because it is easier to perform than spirometry.

In contrast, no single test is 100% sensitive in detecting early COPD and in absence of ideal methods, spirometry together with clinical presentation and history of smoking are the best ways of detecting and confirming COPD. Confirmation of the diagnosis by spirometry and bronchodilator reversibility is the recommended method of early detection, as well as offering a simple means of assessing the extent of disease progression (NICE, 2004).

## How to perform spirometry

Before conducting a reversibility spirometry test, make sure the patient has not used short-acting bronchodilators for at least 6 hours, long-acting bronchodilators for 12 hours and theophylline for 24 hours.

Ideally the test should be conducted when standing, but patients can be seated if required (in case they experience any faintness or syncope during the procedure or for elderly patients who may be unsteady on their feet). Begin by explaining the purpose of the test. Explain the correct procedure and if necessary demonstrate it to them. Ask the patient to blow out so that maximal inhalation occurs. Encourage the patient to keep blowing out so that maximal exhalation can be achieved. Limit the total number of attempts (practice and for recording) to eight or less at each session and record the best of three for calculation purposes.

### Practical hints

Criteria for satisfactory blows are:

1 The blow should continue until a volume plateau is reached – this may take more than 12 seconds in severe COPD. Some devices may bleep twice to indicate the process is complete.
2 FVC and $FEV_1$ readings should be within 5% or 100 mL.
3 The expiratory volume–time graph should be smooth and free from irregularities.

| Table 9.2 Reversibility test | | |
|---|---|---|
| **Bronchodilator** | **Asthma** | **FEV₁ before and after** |
| Salbutamol | 2.5–5 mg (nebuliser)<br>200–400 µg (large-volume spacer) | 20 minutes |
| Terbutaline | 5–10 mg (nebuliser)<br>500 µg (large-volume spacer) | 20 minutes |
| Ipratropium bromide | 500 µg (nebuliser)<br>160 µg (large-volume spacer) | 45 minutes |
| From Bellamy *et al.*, 2005. Reproduced with permission from the British Thoracic Society. | | |

Complete pre-dose spirometry and, after administering the required dose of bronchodilators, ask the patient to wait for the required time and perform post-dose spirometry according to the description in *Table 9.2*. Reversibility can also be completed following the administration of either oral or inhaled corticosteroids therapy. In the case of oral therapy, a pre-dose spirometry followed by post-spirometry after two weeks of oral dosing with 30-40mg prednisolone is obtained.

With a corticosteroid inhaler, patients are given 1000µg daily for three months before post-spirometry is completed. In any case, an increase of 20% in FEV1 or 400ml would indicated asthma.

An increase in $FEV_1$ of >15% or >200 mL from baseline is significant. An increase of >20% and >400 mL is suggestive of asthma.

## Case studies

### Case study 1

Mr SZ, a 54-year-old man, was first seen about six months ago for COPD evaluation. At the time he appeared to be anxious and depressed, although computer records pointed to discontinuation of the medication due to non-compliance with antidepressant. Clinical diagnosis of COPD was made 4 years ago. This was based on recurrent chest infections (bronchitis) and a long history of cigarette smoking since the age of 13. The patient stopped smoking about 5 years ago.

Depression is very common amongst patients with established COPD. NICE recommends regular assessment for any signs of depression and immediate treatment when depression is confirmed. If depression is suspected, treat if within your competency otherwise refer to another healthcare professional.

Smoking status should be recorded each time the patient is consulted and where the patient is a smoker, smoking cessation should be encouraged and offered.

There was no record of any spirometric investigation to confirm the clinical diagnosis of COPD. The symptoms mainly consisted of an increase in sputum production, shortness of breath, wheezy at times, early morning chest congestion and gradual deterioration in breathing ability that got worse during cold season. He denied having asthma, had no allergic hay fever, family history of asthma or childhood eczema. Symptoms appeared to worsen with time, although they had improved since he stopped smoking. His father apparently was a heavy smoker and died of unknown cause. It is unclear if his father's smoking habit was the cause of his medical condition. Although Mr SZ stopped smoking 5 years ago, it was necessary to remind him of further risks if he started to smoke again. The patient was adamant that he would never smoke again.

He appeared to have nasal congestion, apparently a permanent feature of his symptoms, which appeared to be continuous in nature. Although he was given antihistamines in the past, he never complied with them.

His medications included salbutamol inhaler to be used when required and beclometasone 200 µg twice daily. Computer records for prescriptions issued for beclometasone and salbutamol revealed non-compliance with the former and over-compliance with the latter medication. The patient confirmed that he rarely used beclometasone because it did not do anything to relieve symptoms and he was very much dependent on salbutamol for symptom relief.

Non-compliance with inhaled corticosteroids is very common among asthmatic and COPD patients. This is partly due to a lack of understanding of the inhaler's properties. Furthermore, device suitability for individual patients appears to play an important role in treatment failure. Guidelines suggest agreeing concordance with the patients and checking the inhaler technique at every consultation and follow-up.

Asthma is very common among those with allergic rhinitis and to this end British Thoracic Society (2008) guidelines recommend exclusion of rhinitis before fully treating a patient's asthma. The existence of triggering factors such as pollen, house dust mites, animal fur (e.g. cats and dogs), viral infections and chemical irritants lends support to the confirmation of asthma in individual patients. Triggering factors are mainly allergic in nature, although irritants can cause reactions by simply irritating the already inflamed airways.

Asthmatic patients with atopy produce excessive amounts of immunoglobulin E (IgE), which is triggered by allergens such as pollen, house dust mites or animal fur. Individuals with atopy have a genetic predisposition to produce IgE antibodies against common environmental allergens. It has been suggested that those with an allergic component will go on to develop atopic dermatitis early in life, which in some cases will settle down and in others will progress and develop into allergic rhinitis, asthma or both

(Spergel and Paller, 2003). The evidence to support allergic rhinitis as a risk factor for developing asthma is overwhelming. A threefold increase in asthma incidence in patients with allergic rhinitis has been suggested (Settipane *et al.*, 1994; Skoner, 2000; British Thoracic Society, 2008).

The mechanism by which rhinitis leads to asthma incidence is thought to involve the release of cytokines and chemokines into the circulation following stimulation by the allergens. These enter the bone marrow and cause production of white blood cells, in particular eosinophils. The influx of eosinophils into upper and lower airways causes inflammation, hyperactivity of smooth muscle and contractions, hence causing an asthma attack (Burns, 2007).

### Discussion

The NICE guideline recommends the use of spirometric evaluation to confirm diagnoses of COPD and a reversibility test to exclude asthma as the cause of respiratory symptoms that are common in both asthma and COPD (NICE, 2004). Because the patient already had a clinical diagnosis of COPD on his record, he should be given a spirometry test to confirm the initial diagnosis.

The spirometry test revealed very severe obstruction. The reversibility test was scheduled to take place in two weeks' time to see if the obstruction could be reversed.

Some spirometers automatically generate graphs together with the interpretation of the results. The severity of the obstruction is determined by the $FEV_1$ value. COPD is graded based on the patient performance in producing results, in particular $FEV_1$ (*Table 9.3*). $FEV_1$ is the volume of expelled air in the first second of a forced expiration. This is normally reduced in both obstructive and restrictive lung disease.

The guideline also recommends that the treatments should be based on the initial diagnosis, in this case COPD, unless superseded by asthma on the reversibility test. For this reason, the patient was initially given a treatment regimen that was more suitable for a COPD condition.

Because of the severity of the symptoms and the degree of obstruction, based on NICE guidelines, use of a high-dose steroid with a long-acting beta-agonist is considered beneficial in symptomatic patients.

**Table 9.3** The degree of obstruction based on NICE and British Thoracic Society guidelines

| | |
|---|---|
| $FEV_1$ >80% of predicted | COPD unlikely (no obstruction) |
| $FEV_1$ 50–80% of predicted | Mild airflow obstruction |
| $FEV_1$ 30–49% of predicted | Moderate airflow obstruction |
| $FEV_1$ <30% of predicted | Severe airflow obstruction |

A high-dose steroid is reserved for patients with confirmed moderate to severe COPD with two or more exacerbations in the last 12 months (NICE, 2004).

A high-dose inhaler containing 400 µg budesonide and 12 µg formoterol is considered one option in this patient. Other options that are available include a high-dose inhaler containing fluticasone 500 µg and salmeterol 50 µg.

For the purposes of this exercise, the patient was given the 400 µg budesonide/12 µg formoterol high-dose inhaler to be used twice daily. Instructions on how to use the inhaler device and the frequency of dosing were given and concordance with the medications agreed with the patient. To avoid fungal infections of the mouth or the throat and systemic absorption of the high-dose steroid, the patient should be instructed to rinse his mouth out with a glass of water every time he uses the steroid inhaler.

Mr SZ was asked to return for a reversibility test. To complete the reversibility test, the patient was given a 400 µg salbutamol inhaler via a spacer device and asked to wait for 15–20 minutes. The subsequent spirometry reversibility test revealed fully reversible obstruction with an increase of 63% in $FEV_1$, 40% in $FEV_1/FVC$ ratio and significant increases in all other respiratory parameters compared with the pre-dose test. The computer record provided insight into previous records of PEFR, which should be used as the baseline for future PEFR monitoring.

According to the NICE guideline (2004) on the treatment of COPD, an increase of more that 20% in $FEV_1$ would be indicative of asthma. For this reason, the initial diagnosis of COPD should no longer be valid and needs further review. It was clear that the patient suffered from asthma and that COPD was not a dominant feature of his symptoms. With this new development, the treatment regimen that was adopted at the early stage of diagnosis was in need of change.

As described earlier, personal or family history of asthma or atopy (eczema, allergic rhinitis) lends support to diagnosis of asthma in an individual person affected by the asthma symptoms. Although this patient had no family history, it appeared that he may be suffering from allergic rhinitis. One feature of his symptoms that points to possible allergic component was the presence of ongoing nasal blockage and nasal drips. Apart from non-compliance with corticosteroid inhaler therapy, nasal symptoms could be considered a possible cause of uncontrolled asthma and the reason for frequent episodes of exacerbation. The patient's cough appeared to have elements of infective phlegm, which could be secondary to allergic rhinitis, especially since the reversibility tests excluded the presence of a COPD condition.

It is therefore safe to assume that any reduction in degree of exposure to these triggering factors, as mentioned earlier, will ultimately result in reduction in severity, and help to prevent exacerbations and the need to use high doses of medications for symptom control. Therefore it is important to evaluate the triggering factors leading to uncontrolled asthma once the diagnosis of asthma is confirmed (British Thoracic Society, 2008). Giving the patient an atopy test would confirm diagnosis.

The decision to include beclometasone nasal spray in conjunction with regular anti-inflammatory inhaler therapy should be taken to treat allergic rhinitis and reduce the impact on asthma. In theory recurrent chest infections and acute episodes of exacerbations could be reduced if rhinitis is fully controlled and treated. Steroid nasal sprays are an effective method of allergic rhinitis treatment (Burns, 2007; NHS Prodigy, 2008). Oral antihistamines are also used to treat the condition, but because the patient did not respond well to oral antihistamine therapy, nasal steroids appeared to be a better option. In some cases both oral antihistamine and steroid nasal spray are used to control symptoms.

Follow-up appointments provided further clues and supported the diagnosis of asthma in conjunction with allergic rhinitis. Recently, the patient was treated for severe exacerbation following spring cleaning of his house. Apparently, he was exposed to overwhelming dust while cleaning and consequently sought emergency consultation. High-dose prednisolone (30 mg daily) for 7 days apparently helped the new episode of exacerbation. This episode occurred after a long period of stability while he was compliant with his asthma medications: 400 µg budesonide/12 µg formoterol high-dose inhaler and beclometasone nasal spray. It appears that the Mr SZ might be allergic to house dust mites rather than pollen.

Although the 400 µg budesonide/12 µg formoterol high-dose inhaler is used to treat both asthma and COPD, the treatment approach between the two conditions is different. Because of the symptoms' variability, allergic nature and causes of asthma, steroid inhalers form the mainstay of treatment, allowing stepping up when uncontrolled and stepping down the treatment when the condition is stabilised. In contrast, in COPD, trials of high-dose steroids are used when initial therapies fail to control symptoms in those with moderate to severe obstruction with recurrent exacerbation.

The 400 µg budesonide/12 µg formoterol high-dose inhaler was primarily used to treat COPD, as the initial assessment suggested, but following confirmation of asthma, this was downgraded gradually to lower dose of 200/6 µg to be used twice daily. This decision was taken when the patient's PEFR was stabilised at 500 L/min.

A gradual dose reduction of 50% in inhaled steroid therapy in asthmatic patients after three months of complete control is suggested (British Thoracic Society, 2008). Regular asthma reviews must be planned and further support given when needed. All patients should be provided with an asthma treatment plan so that exacerbations and emergency admissions can be avoided.

The reduction in dose had no adverse effect on asthma control. The patient appeared to have fully controlled asthma at this stage.

Beclometasone nasal spray appeared to mostly reverse the continuous nose block, mucosal nasal swelling and nasal drips. Further reduction in steroid therapy was planned three months after the last medication review. The budesonide/formoterol inhaler was further reduced to 100/6 µg to be used twice daily and again the asthma stayed fully controlled on the lower maintenance dose.

Peak expiratory flow rate (PEFR) should be used to monitor the effectiveness of any given treatment. This can be used to instruct the patient to step-up as well as step-down the treatment (British Thoracic Society, 2008).

The PEFR stayed at the same level as before. When questioned at this stage he stated that he had not used salbutamol for at least three months while using regular steroid inhaler.

This case illustrates the adverse effects of allergens on asthma control and potential exacerbations resulting from these. It is also worth mentioning that the peak flow measure before initiating the new regimen was 240 L/min. This increased to 380 L/min following initial monotherapy with the budesonide/formoterol inhaler and further increased to 550 L/min when beclometasone nasal spray was added to the regimen.

Allergen avoidance measures may be helpful in reducing the severity of existing disease and exacerbation in some patients (NHS Prodigy, 2008). Pollen avoidance measures that are recommended to improve the management of asthma or reduced exacerbations include, use of pollen filters in cars, avoiding open grassy spaces, especially in the evening, and closure of windows during high pollen seasons (Roberts, 2002; British Thoracic Society, 2008).

House dust mites are more difficult to eradicate and it is very expensive to carry out complete mite eradication, rendering this method ineffective in the prophylactic treatment of asthma (Gotzsche and Johansen, 1998). The available evidence does not support use of such methods because of the cost involved and indicates that such a measure may not be beneficial in all cases (British Thoracic Society, 2008), although in some cases where all measures have failed to help with symptom control or in cases where there is personal preference in adopting such a measure, control of house dust mites using a number of measures may be beneficial and effective.

Bearing this in mind, this patient should be educated on future house cleaning activities and advised to use a dust-removing mask, high filtration vacuum cleaners designed to contain dust and the use of wet cloths to collect dust if such activities are carried out in the future.

Non-compliance with steroid-based inhaler therapy is the major cause of poor asthma control (British Thoracic Society, 2008). There are a number of factors involved with non-compliance with inhaler therapies, some medication related and others non-medication related. These include, lack of knowledge about the medications, lack of knowledge of the need to take regular anti-inflammatory medications, concerns with long-term usage (specially parental concerns with growth retardation), patient perception of his or her disease state, fear of side-effects, difficulty using inhaler devices, awkward treatment regimens, lack of guidance for self-management, dissatisfaction with healthcare professionals, poor supervision, training or follow-up and cultural issues.

Factors that led to Mr SZ's non-compliance with anti-inflammatory inhaler medications were lack of knowledge about the properties of anti-inflammatory medication, difficulty using the inhaler device, lack of guidance on self-management, lack of medication reviews and follow-ups and concerns with long-term usage of anti-inflammatory inhalers. Mr SZ was fearful that his body would develop tolerance if he used long-term steroids. He had no insight into the properties of steroid inhalers and was not aware that if it is used regularly it would prevent attacks or reduce frequencies of exacerbation.

For asthma to be treated effectively and successfully, one must rely on the patients' cooperation with instruction and compliance with the medications. It is therefore important to fully engage with the patient at all stages of consultation.

To improve the patient–healthcare professional's relationship one must be prepared to listen to patient's beliefs and concerns, allow enough time for patients to ask questions and provide information when needed.

Effective patient education has been shown to improve compliance (Levy *et al.*, 2000; Morice and Wrench, 2000; Newell, 2006), achieve clinical outcomes (British Thoracic Society, 2008; Jewitt, 2001), reduced exacerbation, hospitalisation and improved self-management (Levy *et al.*, 2000).

A survey looking at outcomes of asthma treatment in children (Rabe *et al.*, 2000) found that 34% of patients (or parents) were unaware that inflammation was the underlying condition of asthma. The same study also revealed that 72% of patients believed there is a strong need for better patient education, with only 9% of patients reporting having received a written asthma action plan.

A written self-managed asthma action plan, when provided, has been shown to reduce emergency hospital admissions and emergency GP consultations, and to save lives and money (Levy *et al.*, 2000; NICE, 2004; British Thoracic Society, 2006).

Action plans, where provided, are viewed positively by patients (Douglas *et al.*, 2002). A self-managed action plan is an agreement between the patient and a healthcare professional. The plan deals with the steps the patient can take when asthma symptoms deteriorate or if the patient has fully gained control of an otherwise uncontrolled asthma. It allows the patient stepping-up treatment as well as stepping-down to achieve maximum benefit, reduce symptoms, reduce dose where justified and avoid emergency admissions. It is estimated that approximately 20% of adults and 28% of children seek an unscheduled emergency visit to a healthcare professional at least once a year (National Asthma Campaign, 2001). In 2006, in the UK, well over 1300 patients died from asthma (British Thoracic Society, 2006); the figure being highest among children and vulnerable elderly patients.

From the consultation point of view, Mr SZ was symptomatic, had had a number of exacerbations and emergency consultations, he was non-compliant with asthma medications, his knowledge of his disease condition was minimal, he did not know how and when to use his inhalers, he was unaware of the underlying inflammatory component to his asthma, he rarely had an asthma review and had a very poor inhaler technique.

The structured consultations should provide opportunities to review patients' medications, reinforce and extend patients' knowledge and skills, provide education on the reality of living with asthma, explain future implications of non-compliance with preventative medications, explain the underlying cause, and obtain a consensus and agreed action plan.

The patient was given a written action plan that allowed him to step up as well as step down his treatment regimen.

The action plan should cover the dosage regimen for preventative medications, when to recognise changes in symptoms, duration of dose increase (stepping up), when to reduce (stepping down) and how and when to seek medical attention.

An example of a typical action plan that can be provided to patients is shown in *Table 9.4*. The action plan uses a combination of objective assessments and severity of symptoms to provide guidance on the course of action that the patient needs to take.

This action plan is based on the outcome of recent studies looking at exacerbations and degree of asthma control (Aalbers *et al.*, 2004; Vogelmeier *et al.*, 2005). Aalbers *et al.* showed that patients who are given adjustable budesonide/formoterol dosing are 40% less likely to experience severe exacerbation (defined as exacerbations requiring oral steroid treatment for at least 3 days, emergency home visit or hospitalisation) than those who were given fixed doses of budesonide/formoterol or salmeterol/fluticasone. The adjustable budesonide/formoterol also provided significantly superior asthma control (less bronchial dilator usage, peak flow measurements) than fixed dosing with other regimens. The author of the study concluded that for every 100 patients switched from fixed dose to adjustable dose, 20 less patients would be prevented from being affected by severe exacerbation in one year. The cost saving due to reduced hospitalisation was considered significant.

In the study by Vogelmeier *et al.* (2005), when budesonide/formoterol was used as both maintenance and reliever, the risk of severe asthma attack

| Table 9.4 Typical asthma action plan | | |
|---|---|---|
| **Peak expiratory flow rate (your personal best: 550 L/min** | **Symptoms** | **Treatment** |
| 550 L/min | Asthma controlled; no symptoms; salbutamol hardly used | Budesonide/formoterol inhaler 100/6 µg: one dose twice daily. Salbutamol when needed |
| >250–400 L/min | Waking up at night at least once or twice weekly; occasional wheeze; more than twice weekly salbutamol use | Budesonide/formoterol inhaler 100/6 µg: two doses twice daily and additional doses added if symptomatic; up to two extra doses twice daily until peak flows are back to your personal best for 3 consecutive days. If after the first day, despite using additional dose, the peak flow has stayed low, make an emergency appointment with your GP. The extra doses can be used any time you have symptoms (i.e. 10 minutes or more after your morning and evening doses). If not able to recover from acute attack despite using extra doses, seek emergency consultation with your GP. Salbutamol when needed |
| <250 L/min | Shortage of breath; wheeze and cough; frequently waking up with asthma | Return to surgery for emergency consultation. Insist on seeing your GP on the same day. Follow above regimen until you are seen by your doctor |
| <180 L/min | Severe attack not responding to inhalers; unable to speak because of attack | Don't wait – go straight to A&E |

in this group of patients reduced by 25% and the number of asthma attacks by 23%, in comparison to those patients who used salmeterol/fluticasone and short-acting bronchial dilator reliever (salbutamol).

In comparison to salmeterol, formoterol has a rapid onset of action (300 minutes vs 120 minutes), comparable with that of salbutamol (Cazzola *et al.*, 2003). Because of the dose–response properties of formoterol, higher or more frequent doses can be given if symptoms worsen (Canonica *et al.*, 2004).

Treatment of asthma involves a stepwise approach; the initial step involves treatment with a short-acting beta$_2$-agonist such as a salbutamol inhaler. The level of inhaler therapy increases with increase in severity, leading to the second step of therapy involving a short-acting beta$_2$-agonist and steroid therapy given via an inhalation device. The aims of drug therapy are to control asthma symptoms (whether nocturnal or exercise induced), avoid exacerbations and achieve a near normal lung function for individual patients (British Thoracic Society, 2008).

Monotherapy with either short-acting or long-acting beta$_2$-agonists is not recommended because studies in asthma patients have shown an increase in mortality, especially among children (Hasford and Virchow, 2006). A similar outcome has been seen in COPD patients (Calverley, 2006). For this reason British Thoracic Society (2008) guidelines recommend the use of corticosteroid or corticosteroid/beta$_2$-agonist combined medication in all asthma patients. Steroids are the drugs of choice because they treat inflammation; the underlying cause of asthma.

Although the maintenance dose used by Mr SZ was less than those used in these two studies, the patient appeared to respond very well to the devised regimen and in nine months experienced no exacerbation except when he carried out spring cleaning of his house, at which point the inhalers failed to fully control the symptoms. Peak flow during this episode of exacerbation fell to 250 L/min (by more than half the personal best) before he sought emergency consultation with his GP. The action plan appeared to work for him at every stage. His use of the salbutamol inhaler during the period of stability was absolutely minimal (one inhaler in nine months) compared with two or more per months before any action was taken.

## Case study 2

Mrs ZZ attended a hypertension clinic in 2007. She was considered an infrequent visitor to the surgery. The last medication review for her was in 1998, when she was seen for acute cough and shortness of breath. Examination at the time revealed hypertension (210/90 mmHg) together with clinical diagnosis of COPD, which was mainly based on clinical symptoms and continual smoking since the age of 13. There was no spirometric confirmation of this condition either at the time of consultation or at any time in the following years. Further examination of computer files revealed that the patient had had a number of episodes of chest infections and exacerbations, for which antibiotics and steroids were prescribed. Further consultation revealed that Mrs ZZ had experienced an increase in sputum production in recent years, with gradual deterioration in her breathing ability. Mrs ZZ preferred self-medication and therefore went to her local pharmacy every time she developed a cough. On occasions, she would come to the surgery if symptoms persisted beyond a few days of self-treatment.

Her medications consisted of salbutamol/ipratropium bromide inhaler, which she found most helpful in relieving dyspnoea and shortness of breath, although this was not fully effective in complete respiratory symptom relief. Other medications included antihypertensives including captopril and simvastatin.

Mrs ZZ was encouraged to stop smoking but this was last in Mrs ZZ's list of priorities because she felt it was the only enjoyment she had and she would have liked to continue smoking. We agreed never to raise this issue again. Mrs ZZ continues to smoke to date.

Smoking cessation is the only intervention that is considered to be beneficial in COPD patients. Smoking cessation should be encouraged at every stage (Calverley, 2006; NICE, 2004).

Beside diagnosis of COPD, Mrs ZZ had other co-morbidities, which required further attention. Her blood pressure was raised on three occasions (180/90 to 210/90) despite the fact that she was taking the maximum dose of captopril. Priority was placed on controlling blood pressure before any action was taken in COPD symptom control. When the patient complained of a persistent irritating non-productive cough lasting for three weeks, her antihypertensive medication was reviewed. Blood pressure was raised at the time of consultation. Captopril was discontinued and replaced with valsartan to exclude cough associated with an ACE inhibitor. Chest infection was excluded following physical examination. Amlodipine and bendroflumethiazide were added to the valsartan, in order to optimise blood pressure. Following that intervention, the patient's blood pressure stabilised between 140/70 and 150/80 mmHg.

A persistent irritating cough lasting more than two weeks in patients on ACE inhibitors may indicate side-effects associated with the medication and should not be confused with worsening of the COPD. Detailed consultation and chest examination should differentiate between the two.

Overall, 22% of patients with mild to moderate COPD may die from cardiovascular causes. It is therefore imperative to detect and identify COPD patients at an early stage, so that those with highest risk of overall mortality from cardiovascular and ischaemic heart disease can be detected, monitored and effectively treated.

Treating co-morbidities is as important as treating the COPD itself, because it has been established that patients with COPD die from causes other than respiratory failure. In a study by Anthonisen *et al.* (2005), which followed patients for 14 years with mild to moderate COPD, 22% of patients died because of cardiovascular events. In a separate study (Anthonisen *et al.*, 2002) the rate of hospitalisation in COPD patients due to cardiovascular events was 42–48%, with only 14% hospitalised for acute exacerbation of COPD. Considering the above, it was vitally important to treat Mrs ZZ's hypertension at the earliest opportunity, before attempting to optimise drug treatment of COPD. Because of the nature of the patient's disease state, caution should be exercised so that drug–disease interactions can be avoided. For this reason beta-blockers are contraindicated in asthma and used with great caution in COPD patients.

Review of COPD started when Mrs ZZ developed further acute exacerbation of chest symptoms. Mrs ZZ was prescribed a short course of oral prednisolone 30 mg taken daily. The treatment improved Mrs ZZ's symptoms.

It is best practice to postpone any spirometric investigation following acute exacerbation until full recovery is achieved.

Pharmaceutical interventions mainly involved the use of inhaled medications, with occasional oral medications to alleviate severity of the disease. Most of the lung function impairment in COPD patients is fixed, although some reversibility can be produced by bronchodilator (or other) therapies (British Thoracic Society, 1997; NICE, 2004).

The aims of therapy for COPD are to prevent disease progression, relieve symptoms, increase self-confidence, prevent and treat complications and exacerbations, reduce morbidity and mortality. Despite all the efforts, COPD is the third highest respiratory killer, overtaking death caused by ischaemic heart disease (British Thoracic Society, 2006).

NICE (2004) guidelines suggest a stage-wise approach in treatment of patients with COPD. In stage 1, a short-acting bronchodilator (beta$_2$-agonist or anticholinergic), used as necessary, is the initial empirical treatment for the relief of breathlessness and exercise limitation. The patient should be assessed for the effectiveness of the treatment using lung function and a variety of other measures such as improvement in symptoms, activities of daily living, exercise capacity, and rapidity of symptom relief.

In stage 2, combined therapy with a short-acting beta$_2$-agonist and a short-acting anticholinergic, with or without long-acting bronchodilators, should be used in patients who are still symptomatic. Long-acting bronchodilators (beta$_2$-agonist and tiotropium; anticholinergics) should be used in patients who remain symptomatic or who have had two or more exacerbations per year, despite treatment with combined short-acting bronchodilators.

In stage 3, a combination of short-acting and long-acting bronchodilators may be used together with high-dose steroid therapy if the patient is still symptomatic and has moderate to severe obstruction on spirometry with two or more exacerbations per year. Treatment may include theophylline in those who still show signs and symptoms of the disease.

Evidence for use of inhaled medications comes from number of randomised and unrandomised cross-over clinical trials. The choice of drug(s) will depend on patient's preference, device suitability and response to a trial of the drug, cost and side-effects of the prescribed medication (NICE, 2004).

In one study Macie *et al.* (2006) examined 90–365-day mortality rates following hospital discharge, and concluded that when steroid inhalers are given 30 days post discharge, survival rates were significantly higher in the steroid group than in those who received long-acting beta$_2$-agonists or nothing at all. Furthermore, results from the TORCH (TOwards a Revolution in COPD Health) study (Calverley, 2006) showed a 17% relative reduction in mortality over 3 years for patients who received an inhaler containing fluticasone/salmeterol (50/500 µg) compared with patients on placebo. The combination also reduced the rate of COPD exacerbations by 25% compared to placebo and resulted in an improvement in quality of life when compared to placebo as measured by the St George's Respiratory Questionnaire.

When comparing the combination of fluticasone/salmeterol to budesonide/formoterol in relatively severe COPD patients (Cazzola et al., 2003), both treatments produced a similar response. Both regimens were safe and no differences in terms of efficacy were seen. However, in the budesonide/formoterol group, peak activity was achieved after 120 minutes compared with 300 minutes with the fluticasone/salmeterol group. This is possibly because formoterol has a rapid onset of action, comparable with that of salbutamol, and therefore potentially can be used as a rescue medication. Because of the dose–response properties of formoterol, higher or more frequent doses can be given if symptoms worsen (Canonica et al., 2004).

Combination therapy with formoterol and budesonide was therefore preferred for Mrs ZZ since she fulfils the criteria for high-dose combination therapy.

The NICE (2004) guidelines suggest initiation of high-dose inhaled steroid in patients with moderate to severe obstruction with two or more exacerbations in the last 12 months. Steroid therapy should be reviewed and discontinued if no benefit is gained following the initial therapy.

Some patients may benefit from treatment with theophylline. In one study 33% of patients experienced subjective improvement compared with placebo (Nishimura et al., 1996). However because of the side-effects, the benefits of theophylline in COPD have to be weighed against the risk of adverse effects (Ram et al., 2005).

A long-acting anticholinergic (tiotropium) has been suggested as the second-line treatment of symptomatic patients with COPD, where short-acting bronchodilators fail to control the symptoms (NICE, 2004). The evidence for its use comes from studies that compared tiotropium with salmeterol (Donohue, 2002, Cazzola et al., 2004). Studies have shown that dual combination of long-acting bronchodilators is superior to single agents, and triple therapy with fluticasone is superior to dual-combination or single agents.

It appears that Mrs ZZ is fully controlled and has had no single exacerbation in the last 12 months while on budesonide/formoterol combination therapies and therefore changing the treatment regimen at this time is not warranted. It is planned to prescribe tiotropium if Mrs ZZ's respiratory condition changes in the future. Mrs ZZ is stable at present and a further spirometry test a year later was unchanged.

Treatment of COPD involves pharmacological and non-pharmacological approaches, requiring direct involvement of the patient at all stages. Self-management should form an important part of COPD management strategy. A recent study by Bourbeau et al. (2003) found that the introduction of self-management interventions for patients with COPD significantly reduced the number of admissions for exacerbation and other health problem by 40% and 57%, respectively, and accident and emergency visits by 41%. Overall, there was significant reduction in the utilisation of healthcare services and improvement in the health status of the patient compared with the control group. Unscheduled care accounts for 60% of NHS costs in COPD, mainly from admissions (NICE, 2004) caused by acute exacerbation.

The cost comparison between self-manageed, GP-managed and hospital-managed exacerbations are significantly different; currently estimated as £15, £95 and £1665 per episode respectively (GPIAG, 2005). For this reason the patient was given instructions to return to the surgery when signs and symptoms were indicative of a worsening of the condition. Mrs ZZ was given a peak flow meter to monitor respiratory function (PEFR) and instructed to check the reading against her personal best of 300 L/min. Any reduction below 250 L/min would require an emergency consultation with her GP and reduction below 200 L/min access to an accident and emergency unit.

NICE (2004) recommends that pulse oximetry should be available to all clinicians assessing acute exacerbations. In moderate to severe stable COPD, measurement of blood gas tensions at normal unassisted breathing is recommended. Alternatively, for moderate COPD, measurement of arterial oxygen saturation ($SaO_2$) using a pulse oximeter is sufficient to assure normality. A sequential measurement of blood gas tension becomes necessary if $SaO_2$ value is <92%. Respiratory failure may follow if low oxygen saturation remains low. For this reason Mrs ZZ's oxygen saturation was measured using pulse oximetry, which always gave a reading above 95%.

### Conclusion

One important aspect of treatment of COPD is the direct involvement of the patient in all decision making. Patient education on self-management has been shown to save lives and money. Adherence to local and national guidelines is important. Patients suffering from acute exacerbations should receive prompt assessment, treatment and necessary education to reduce the impact of the disease.

## Case study 3

Amy J, a 4-year-old girl with a family history of asthma, attended an asthma clinic with her father for asthma review. She had been treated for eczema since childhood with emollients and moisturisers.

### Current medications

- Salbutamol inhaler 2 puffs when needed
- Beclometasone inhaler (Qvar) 50 µg 1 puff twice daily

- Montelukast 4 mg chewable tablet every night
- Emollient as required
- Aqueous cream as required.

Amy uses regular salbutamol, sometimes 4–5 times a day and beclometasone only when symptoms are worse. The parents stopped giving montelukast 28 days after it was originally started, because the doctor did not say to continue with the medications. It appeared to help with the symptoms but it did not fully suppress the symptoms. The inhalers are given via an aerochamber spacer with an infant mask attachment. She has been using the chamber since it was first prescribed 2 years ago. She could get breathless when playing with other children. Her father is worried that his daughter having too many asthma attacks in recent weeks and wants your opinion on this and whether something can be done.

She frequently wheezes and quickly develops shortness of breath which responds to salbutamol fairly quickly. In some instances, symptoms are very mild but, can deteriorate rapidly to a more severe asthma attack within 2 hours. On one occasion the attack lasted longer than normal but she was okay.

In the past few weeks, she has developed a cough, mainly at night. This has affected her sleep pattern. Salbutamol inhaler appears to help the cough. Beclometasone was given by her GP about three months ago. This was followed by a prescription for montelukast when she was seen again for follow-up.

Diagnosis of asthma in children is a clinical one and characterised by the presence of more than one symptom including wheeze, cough (mainly early morning/night-time), chest tightness and difficulty breathing. The latest statistics from the British Thoracic Society (2006) indicate that over 1500 patients a year die of a severe acute asthma attack, the majority being children and the elderly.

The presentation of symptoms in children may sometimes indicate other respiratory conditions than asthma. The episodes of wheeze, cough and difficulty breathing are very common in pre-school children who develop viral upper respiratory infections which pass without becoming chronic in nature. A minority of those who develop viral wheeze will go on to become asthmatic with other triggering factors (British Thoracic Society, 2008).

This patient appears to have all the symptoms associated with the asthma condition. Furthermore, asthma is very likely if there is a family history of asthma or atopy (father is asthmatic) and personal history of atopic disorders (eczema in this case). In general, children with asthma will respond very well to adequate medications, whereas in those who are considered non-respondent, diagnosis needs to be revisited and reconfirmed.

One distinct feature of allergic asthma is the occurrence of late response (late phase) following the initial attack (immediate phase). As in Amy's case the late phase occurs one or more hours after the initial phase. The late phase tends to be more troublesome, lasts longer and tends to be severe in nature.

Use of an inhaled steroid in the initial phase can reduce the severity of the late phase in those who have allergic asthma. Providing an asthma action plan to incorporate extra doses of inhaled steroid would be beneficial.

Because of the history and nature of symptoms, one can safely diagnose allergic asthma in this case. The fact that she responds to treatment when given indicates that her asthma can be treated easily. It appears that the underlying cause in Amy's case is atopic asthma leading to inflammation.

Atopy refers to a collection of allergic conditions that are IgE mediated and associated with release of IgE autoimmune antibodies causing a wide range of symptoms, including worsening of asthma in susceptible individuals. Allergen avoidance is therefore considered an important component of asthma treatment in those with history of atopy. Allergens that are widely known to precipitate asthma include pollens, house dust mites, some food products (nuts) and fungi. There is also cross-reactivity between tree pollens and some fruit (e.g. patients who have allergy to birch tree pollen may also develop late response allergy to apple and peach). A diary of food intake and late response reactions can eliminate the source of allergies in children.

Diagnosis of asthma in children over the age of 5 and in adults is supported by conventional lung function tests such as spirometry and peak flow (PEFR measurements) and reversibility testing using two devices. In children under the age of 5 these methods have no place and the emphasis is on clinical diagnosis. To manage the condition effectively it is necessary to educate the parents on the asthma condition, the underlying causes and the objectives of the treatments. Frequent wheeze and breathlessness is mainly caused by non-compliance with the medications, a lack of understanding of the causes of asthma and a lack of knowledge about the properties of inhalers.

British Thoracic Society (2008) guidelines on the treatment of asthma suggest trial treatment with inhaled beta$_2$-agonist and corticosteroid therapy, the choice depending on the severity and frequency of symptoms. In this case, compliance with prescribed medication should overcome some if not all of the asthma symptoms. Because the patient is still experiencing frequent attacks despite using salbutamol, a trial addition of corticosteroid would be beneficial. Qvar is not licensed for under 12 years of age and therefore needs to be changed to an alternative CFC-free inhaler, Clenil Modulite 50 µg, using two puffs (100 µg) twice daily or budesonide 100 µg twice daily. The former is an alternative to non-CFC beclometasome inhalers, which are due to be phased out once the existing supplies are exhausted. The British Thoracic Society (2008) suggests brand prescribing of CFC-free beclometasone-containing inhalers to avoid overdosing.

Higher doses of steroids (200–400 μg daily) can be used in children under 5 years of age when a smaller dose is inadequate to fully control the asthma. Once asthma control is achieved, titrate to the lowest dose at which effective control of asthma is maintained.

Before changing the dose or initiating a new inhaled therapy, recheck compliance, inhaler technique and eliminate triggering factors (British Thoracic Society, 2008).

Good asthma control is associated with little or no need for short-acting beta$_2$-agonists such as salbutamol. Using two canisters of salbutamol per month or >10–12 puffs of inhaler per day is an indication of poorly controlled asthma. Inhaled steroids are considered effective preventers if used properly. They are considered if the child has one or more of the following (NICE, 2008):

- exacerbation of asthma in the past 2 years
- using inhaled beta$_2$-agonists three times a week or more
- symptomatic three times a week or more
- waking one night a week.

This patient fulfils all criteria for inhaled corticosteroid therapy. Amy's father was encouraged to give a regular dose of steroid inhaler and record the number of times the salbutamol inhaler is used, episodes of night-time cough and frequency of exacerbation until the next consultation. He was also provided with an action plan to manage exacerbations, coughs and wheeze.

The action plan had the following elements:

- Increase budesonide to 4 puffs twice daily via spacer device if (a) woken-up with cough once per week, (b) salbutamol used more than three times per week, or (c) symptoms worsen suddenly and wheeze develops.
- Then continue with the new treatment and make an appointment to see the GP.
- Seek emergency consultation/accident and emergency admission if standard dose and subsequent doses of salbutamol given via spacer device fails to control the acute asthma attack.

In infants and children, inhaled steroids and other metered dose inhalers are best given via spacer devices. Inhaled beta$_2$-agonist given via volume spacer to mild to moderate asthmatic patients is considered as effective as nebulised solutions (British Thoracic Society, 2008). Spacer devices are required to be cleaned at least once a month, by washing in detergent and allowing to dry in air. The patient had used the spacer for over 2 years and the actual spacer was no longer suitable for her age (infant mask). A new spacer device with a child mask is appropriate, otherwise if the child can manage, a spacer device with mouthpiece is suitable.

Continual and regular usage of budesonide 100 µg twice daily fully controlled Amy's asthma symptoms. The need for salbutamol was completely diminished, although in one instance she needed to use salbutamol more than three times in one day. This coincided with development of one episode of night-time cough once in the last four weeks. Efforts to reduce the budesonide to the lowest possible dose led to increased asthma symptoms. Because the child previously responded to montelukast therapy, it was appropriate to add this to her medications again before attempting to reduce budesonide dose. British Thoracic Society (2008) guidelines suggest addition of leukotriene receptor antagonist (e.g. montelukast) if the maintenance daily dose of steroid is between 200 and 400 µg. This allows steroid dose reduction to lowest possible level.

Patients should start treatment at the step most appropriate to the initial severity of their asthma. Dosage of inhaled steroid should be moved down to find and maintain the lowest controlling step (British Thoracic Society, 2008).

## Conclusion

Evidence available here indicates that Amy may have allergic asthma, triggered by one or more allergens. Non-compliance with steroid therapy is considered the main cause of treatment failure. Checking and rechecking inhaler technique and compliance are important for success of the treatments. Testing for atopic status should be considered.

Positive skin test, blood eosinophilia >4% or raised specific IgE to cat, dog or mite increase the probability of asthma in a child with wheeze (British Thoracic Society, 2008).

## Case study 4

Mrs JA, 59 years old, was referred for spirometry following the development of breathlessness and dyspnoea. The patient stopped smoking after 30 years with a history of 20 pack-years.

### Past and current medical history
- COPD (on clinical presentation)
- Asthma
- Suspected congestive heart failure
- Hypertension
- Hyperlipidaemia.

### Current medications
- Diltiazem 180 mg XL daily
- Furosemide 40 mg two tabs daily (only takes 40 mg daily)

- Simvastatin 40 mg at night
- Combivent inhaler two puffs four times daily
- Seretide Accuhaler 250 µg one dose twice daily

### Clinical presentations

Pale looking, shortness of breath (wakes up with cough few hours after sleep), rapid and shallow breathing, occasional wheeze, pulse oximetry 92% saturation, phlegm present at all times (clear), nocturnal cough, unable to walk more than 20 m (breathless). No ankle swelling or oedema, blood pressure 140/85 mmHg, pulse 76 bpm.

### Investigations

Severe obstruction on spirometric test.

### Diagnosis

- Acute exacerbation of COPD?
- Acute congestive heart failure?

### Discussion

Examination of her medical notes did not produce conclusive evidence for the presence of asthma. The respiratory problem started about 7 years ago, at which time she was given salbutamol inhaler to control breathlessness and night-time cough. The diagnosis of COPD (bronchitis) was made when the patient presented with chest infection. The diagnosis was based on long-term smoking, the presence of continuous phlegm in the chest and the presence of infection.

The current signs and symptoms are suggestive of aggravated congestive cardiac failure or acute COPD exacerbation.

There are distinct differences between asthma, COPD and cardiac asthma. As the name suggests, cardiac asthma refers to respiratory signs and symptoms that are cardiac in origin. Cardiac asthma is caused by failure of the heart to pump the blood around the body. The inefficiency of the left ventricle leads to a build-up of fluid in the lungs (known as pulmonary oedema), causing airways to narrow and wheeze to occur in some cases. The risk of wheeze is greater in those with a history of asthma or COPD. Cardiac asthma shares similar symptoms with bronchial asthma and COPD, although the paths leading to these are different.

The main signs and symptoms of cardiac asthma are:

- shortness of breath with or without wheeze
- cough
- rapid and shallow breathing
- increase pulse rate and blood pressure
- feeling of apprehension.

People with heart failure often wake up after few hours of sleep with shortness of breath and cough, whereas asthmatics wake up with coughing in the early morning. Often, people with bronchial asthma complain of tightness of the chest, whereas this is absent in cardiac asthma (*Table 9.5*).

This is a very complex case that requires input from other healthcare professionals to confirm the diagnosis. The referring GP did not believe the symptoms were caused by heart failure, although some signs such as nocturnal cough (2 hours after going to bed), rapid and shallow breathing and wheeze are suggestive of heart failure. Absence of raised blood pressure, pulse and ankle oedema could be due to administration of diltiazem and furosemide.

**Table 9.5** Clinical features differentiating cardiac asthma, bronchial asthma and COPD

|  | COPD | Bronchial asthma | Cardiac asthma |
|---|---|---|---|
| Smoker or ex-smoker | Nearly all | Possibly | No |
| Symptoms under age 35 years | Rare | Often | Rare |
| Chronic productive cough | Common | Uncommon (may be present with allergic rhinitis) | No |
| Breathlessness | Persistent and progressive | Variable | Variable with degree of heart failure |
| Wheeze | May be present | Present | May be present |
| Breathlessness can develop with: | Slight exertion | Vigorous exertion | Slight or less vigorous exertion |
| Ankle swelling | May be present (end-stage COPD) | Not present | Present if not treated |
| Weight gain | No, some likely to have excessive weight loss | No | Yes. May vary with degree of control/ diuretics therapy |
| Night-time waking with breathlessness and/or wheeze | Uncommon | Common but normally early morning | Common, a few hours after going to bed |
| Significant diurnal or day-to-day variability of symptoms | Uncommon | Common | Uncommon |

In the absence of heart failure, one can attribute the present symptoms to non-infective acute exacerbation of COPD (or asthma), although referral to a cardiologist would be necessary to exclude heart failure as the cause of respiratory symptoms. To exclude asthma, a reversibility test using a short-acting bronchial dilator would be necessary. In the absence of a reversibility test, the patient should be treated for COPD. Before initiation of new therapy, compliance and inhaler techniques should be checked. These were found to be satisfactory.

Like asthma, COPD is treated in a step-wise approach. This patient is currently at stage 3 of the treatment ladder. At stage 3, a combination of short-acting and long-acting bronchodilators may be used together with high-dose steroid therapy, if the patient is still symptomatic and has two or more exacerbations per year. Treatment may include theophylline in those who still show signs and symptoms of the disease. Theophylline has been shown to improve the symptoms associated with both asthma and COPD as well as to significantly increase $FEV_1$ values (Thomas *et al.*, 1992; Nishimura *et al.*, 1996; Tsukino *et al.*, 1998; Ram *et al.*, 2005). In one study 33% of patients experienced subjective improvement compared with placebo (Nishimura, 1996).

Theophylline, like other inhaled agents, relieves symptoms of dyspnoea and cough and acutely improves lung function to some degree, but like other treatments including combinations of long-acting bronchodilators and steroids, it does not modify the long-term decline in $FEV_1$ in COPD patients.

Theophylline has a bronchodilator effect only at a given therapeutic blood level which is between 10–20 mg/L. To achieve this, high doses of theophylline are needed. However, high doses of theophylline can cause a significant degree of nausea and vomiting in normal therapeutic levels and potentially serious life-threatening side-effects if toxic levels present. This means that the benefits of theophylline in COPD have to be weighed against the risk of adverse effects (Ram, 2005).

As mentioned earlier, COPD is a term used to describe the collective symptoms of the lung disease characterised by inflammation of the airway. Once inflammation becomes firmly established, the process persists for many years. With disease progression, the inflammatory process intensifies and becomes more widespread. The inflammation appears to be a neutrophilic in origin (Culpitt, 2002). By subjecting the patients to low-dose theophylline, Culpitt *et al.* (2002) discovered that levels of neutrophils are reduced significantly compared with the control group, suggesting the possibility that low-dose theophylline may be useful in long-term treatment of COPD (Culpitt *et al.*, 2002; Barnes, 2006a, 2006b; Hirano *et al.*, 2006).

A combination of salbutamol, formoterol and theophylline can cause hypokalaemia in elderly patients, especially if a potassium-depleting diuretic such as furosemide is used. Regular urine and electrolyte monitoring is therefore required.

Addition of theophylline to existing medication may also cause hypokalaemia and therefore requires close monitoring. Before initiating theophylline, urine and electrolyte status should be determined unless furosemide is changed to co-amilofruse in which case $K^+$ status needs to be checked regularly.

Because of gastrointestinal side-effects, the theophylline dose should be titrated slowly to a maximum dose of one tablet twice daily after one week.

The addition of theophylline to the patient's medication significantly improved the symptoms, indicating a respiratory element for her symptoms rather than cardiac.

### Conclusion

Patients with heart failure may exhibit symptoms that are very similar to both asthma and COPD. Check drug–drug and drug–disease interactions before initiating new medications. Always involve other healthcare professionals if you have doubt about the working diagnosis. Spirometry is an effective tool in differentiating between asthma, COPD and heart failure.

## Case study 5

James A, a 10-year-old child with a family history of asthma (both parents with history of childhood asthma), attended the asthma clinic for review. Diagnosis of asthma was made at the age of 3, for which salbutamol inhaler was prescribed. James attends boxing training three times a week and is lately finding it difficult to complete boxing activity. There is no personal history of atopy and he denied having other symptoms. He recently started coughing at night time and frequently uses salbutamol to help with the shortness of breath and wheeze. Normally asthma symptoms are relieved after inhaling two puffs of salbutamol, but on one occasion he had to resort to more than six puffs. Frequent wheeze forms part of his symptoms. He does not suffer from a blocked or runny nose.

Computer records indicated that James is non-compliant with inhaled steroid and overcompliant with salbutamol.

Despite having used the inhalers for more than 5 years, James failed to demonstrate good inhalation technique.

### Discussion

It appears that James's asthma is mostly exercise induced, although he can wheeze when not exercising. Night-time cough is an indication of uncontrolled asthma manifested by inflammation as the underlying cause. As with children under age of 5, asthma in children who use frequent salbutamol dosing should be reviewed. The main reason for the high usage of salbutamol is non-compliance with the corticosteroid therapy.

Inhaled steroids are the recommended preventer drug for adults and children for achieving overall treatment goals (British Thoracic Society, 2008). Steroid inhalers are the most effective preventative drugs (Suissa *et al.*, 2002), resulting in better asthma control, reduced hospital admissions and avoiding frequent exacerbation. In some children, as in this case, diagnosis of asthma is made following trial of either a short-acting beta$_2$-agonist or inhaled steroid. The choice of the inhaler depends on the severity and frequency of the symptoms. In general, a positive reaction to either group would indicate the presence of asthma. In children over the age of 5, as in adults, tests of airflow obstruction and airway responsiveness can support the initial diagnosis (British Thoracic Society, 2008).

In children, asthma severity classified by symptoms and measurement of $FEV_1$ in some cases does not correlate with the severity of asthma, whereas measurement of air trapping does correlate better with the severity of asthma and at detecting airway obstruction. In any case, children with a confirmed diagnosis of asthma (spirometry) should be subjected to a reversibility test. An increase of more than 12% in $FEV_1$ or PEFR from baseline confirms reversible airway obstruction and hence a diagnosis of asthma. When James was subjected to spirometry for the first time, this indicated mild obstruction. Reversibility using four puffs (400 µg) of salbutamol inhaler given via large-volume spacer device resulted in a 30% increase in $FEV_1$ value. A large increase in $FEV_1$, indicates responsiveness of the asthma to inhaled steroid. With this in mind, James was educated and instructed to use a steroid inhaler twice daily regularly until he was seen for review in six weeks' time. Because of his poor inhaler technique, he was provided with a small-volume spacer device. He was instructed to keep a diary of asthma events and salbutamol usage.

In children who are considered as having stable asthma, the aim should be to find the minimum effective inhaled steroid dose.

In some cases, it is possible to withdraw steroid treatment after a careful trial of treatment reductions.

As in other cases mentioned here, James was given specific instruction to continue to use a steroid inhaler regularly. The follow-up consultation should incorporate objective lung function measurements such as PEFR and $FEV_1$. Reduced lung function compared with previous measurements may indicate current bronchial constriction or long-term decline in lung function. Continual use of inhaled steroid resulted in lung function normality and further peak flow assessment revealed an increase of 100 L/min from the baseline measurement before the reversibility test. This indicated that James was responding well to the steroid treatment.

Conclusion

In adults and children over the age of 5 years, asthma can be diagnosed using one or more methods such as bronchodilator reversibility testing using spirometry and peak expiratory flow rate measurements. Spirometry is a more reliable method of measurement compared to peak flow rate measurement. An increase of more than 60 L/min in PEF or 12% in $FEV_1$ indicates reversibility and hence confirms diagnosis of asthma.

## Conclusion

Asthma has three distinct elements: symptoms, variable airway obstruction and bronchial hyperresponsiveness. Symptoms consistent with asthma (e.g. wheeze and cough) are also shared by patients with other respiratory diseases, for example by children who contract viral respiratory tract infections or those with COPD, although the latter group exhibit irreversible airways obstruction that does not respond to bronchial dilators. Airways remodelling is a major concern that affects mainly those who are non-compliant with anti-inflammatory medications.

Compliance and concordance with the treatments are the major issues with most asthmatic patients. Effective patient education has been shown to improve compliance and concordance, leading to better clinical outcomes such as reduced exacerbation, improved control and reduced symptoms. One aspect of good asthma management is to provide the patients with a self-managed action plan. This is passively received by the patients and has been shown to save lives and reduce exacerbations and hospital admissions.

Involving the patients in decision making, providing them with necessary information and listening to their beliefs and concerns at all stages of consultation is considered beneficial and affects all aspects of the clinical outcomes in a positive way.

A survey carried out by the Asthma UK Campaign indicates that almost two-thirds of asthma patients are unaware that inflammation is the underlying cause of asthma. Effective education should overcome some of the barriers to successful treatment.

In comparisons between self-managed, GP-managed and hospital-managed exacerbations in COPD patients the costs have been found to be significantly different; currently estimated as £15, £95 and £1665 per episode respectively (GPIAG, 2005). A similar conclusion can be made for exacerbations in asthma patients.

## References

Aalbers R, Backer V, Kava T, Omenaas E R, Sandström T, Jorup C and Welte T (2004). Adjustable maintenance dosing with budesonide/formoterol compared with fixed-dose salmeterol/fluticasone in moderate to severe asthma. *Curr Med Res Opin* 20: 225–240.

Anthonisen N R, Connett J E, Enright P L and Manfreda J (2002). Hospitalizations and mortality in the Lung Health Study. *Am J Respir Crit Care Med*.166: 333–339.

Anthonisen N R, Skeans M A, Wise R A, Manfreda J, Kanner R E and Connett J E (2005). The effects of a smoking cessation intervention on 14.5–year mortality: a randomized clinical trial. *Ann Intern Med*.142: 233–239.

Ball T, Castro-Rodriguez J, Griffith K, Holberg C, Martinez F and Wright A (2000). Siblings, day-care attendance, and the risk of asthma and wheezing during childhood. *N Engl J Med* 343: 538–543.

Barnes P J (2006a). ABC of chronic obstructive pulmonary disease: future treatments. *BMJ* 333: 246–248.

Barnes P J (2006b). Theophylline for COPD: reinstatement in the light of new evidence. *Thorax* 61: 742–743.

Bellamy D, Booker R, Connellan S and Halpin D (2005). Spirometry in practice: a practical guide to using spirometry in primary care. British Thoracic Society (BTS) COPD Consortium. http://www.brit-thoracic.org.uk/Portals/0/Clinical%20Information/COPD/COPD%20 Consortium/spirometry_in_practice051.pdf (accessed 15 April 2009).

Bourbeau J, Julien M, Maltais F, Rouleau M, Beaupré A, Bégin R, Renzi P, Nault D, Borycki E, Schwartzman K, Singh R and Collet J P (2003). Reduction of hospital utilization in patients with chronic obstructive pulmonary disease: a disease-specific self-management intervention. *Arch Intern Med* 163: 585–591.

British Thoracic Society (BTS) (1997). Guidelines for the management of chronic obstructive pulmonary disease. *Thorax* 52 (suppl 5): 521–528.

British Thoracic Society (BTS) (2006). The burden of lung disease: a statistics report from British Thoracic Society, 2nd edn. http://www.erpho.org.uk/Download/Public/15381/1/ BurdenLungDisease2006.pdf (accessed 10 December 2007).

British Thoracic Society and Scottish Intercollegiate Guidelines Network (2008). British guideline on the management of asthma: a national clinical guideline. http://www.brit-thoracic. org.uk/Portals/0/Clinical%20Information/Asthma/Guidelines/asthma_final2008.pdf

Burns D (2007). Management of patients with asthma and allergic rhinitis. *Nurs Stand* 21(26): 48–58.

Calverley P (2006). TORCH findings support combination therapy for COPD. *Pulmonary Reviews*. http://www.pulmonaryreviews.com/dec06/torch.html (accessed 01 December 2007).

Canonica G W, Castellani P, Cazzola M, Fabbri L M, Fogliani V, Mangrella M, Moretti A, Paggiaro P, Sanguinetti C M and Vignola A M (2004). The CAST (Control of Asthma by Symbicort Turbohaler) Study Group. Adjustable maintenance dosing with budesonide/ formoterol in a single inhaler provides effective asthma symptom control at a lower dose than fixed maintenance dosing. *Pulm Pharmacol Ther* 17: 239–247. http://www.ncbi.nlm. nih.gov/entrez/query.fcgi?cmd=retrieve&db=pubmed&list_uids=15219269&dopt=Abst ract (accessed 10/12/2007).

Cazzola M, Santus P, Di Marco F, Boveri B, Castagna F, Carlucci P, Matera MG and Centanni S (2003). Bronchodilator effect of an inhaled combination therapy with salmeterol + fluti-casone and formoterol + budesonide in patients with COPD. *Respir Med*. 97: 453–457.

Cazzola M, Centanni S, Santus P, Verga M, Mondoni M, di Marco F, Matera M G (2004). The functional impact of adding salmeterol and tiotropium in patients with stable COPD. *Respir Med* 98: 1214–1221.

Culpitt S V, de Matos C, Russell R E, Donnelly L E, Rogers D F and Barnes P J (2002). Effect of theophylline on induced sputum inflammatory indices and neutrophil chemotaxis in chronic obstructive pulmonary disease. *Am J Respir Crit Care Med* 165: 1371–1376.

Dezateux C, Stocks J, Dundas I and Fletcher M E (1999). Impaired airway function and wheezing in infancy: the influence of maternal smoking and a genetic predisposition to asthma. *Am J Respir Crit Care Med* 159: 403–410.

Donohue J F, Bateman E D, Lee A, Kesten S, van Noord J A, Langley S J, Witek T J and Tows L (2002). A 6-month, placebo-controlled study comparing lung function and health status changes in COPD patients treated with tiotropium or salmeterol. *Chest* 122: 47–55.

Douglas J, Aroni R, Goeman D, Stewart K, Sawyer S, Thien F and Abramson M (2002). A qualitative study of action plans for asthma. *BMJ* 324: 1003–1007.

Gotzsche P C and Johansen H K (2008). House dust mite control measures for asthma. *Cochrane Database Syst Rev* (2): CD001187.

Gotzsche P C, Hammarquist C and Burr M (1998). House dust mite control measures in the management of asthma: meta-analysis. *BMJ* 317: 1105–1110.

GPIAG (General Practice Airways Group) (2005). Diagnosis and management of chronic obstructive pulmonary disease in primary care: a guide for those working in primary care. http://www.gpiag.org/news/copd_guide/guidelinev14.pdf (accessed 10 December 2007).

Hasford J and Virchow J C (2006). Excess mortality in patients with asthma on long-acting beta$_2$-agonists. *Eur Respir J* 28: 900–902.

Hirano T, Yamagata T, Gohda M, Yamagata Y, Ichikawa T, Yanagisawa S, Ueshima K, Akamatsu K, Nakanishi M, Matssunaga K, Minakata Y and Ichinose M (2006). Inhibition of reactive nitrogen species production in COPD airways: comparison of inhaled corticosteroid and oral theophylline. *Thorax* 61: 761–766.

Jeffery P (1998). Structural and inflammatory changes in COPD: a comparison with asthma. *Thorax* 53: 129–136.

Jewitt K (2001). Staying in control of asthma. *Primary Health Care* 11: 18–20.

Koppelman G H, Jansen D F, Schouten J P, Van der Heide S, Bleecker E R, Meyers D A and Postma D S (2001). Sibling effect on atopy in children of patients with asthma. In: Koppelman G H, ed. *Genetics of Asthma and Atopy*. Baarn: Cordon Art, pp. 83–94. http://dissertations.ub.rug.nl/FILES/faculties/medicine/2001/g.h.koppelman/c4.pdf (accessed 10 January 2008).

Levy M L, Allen J, Doherty C, Bland J M and Winter R J D (2000). A randomized controlled evaluation of specialist nurse education following accident and emergency department attendance for acute asthma. *Respir Med* 94: 900–908.

Lokke A, Lange P, Scharling H, Fabricius P and Vestbo J (2006). Developing COPD: a 25 year follow up study of the general population. *Thorax* 61: 935–939.

Macie C, Wooldrage K, Manfreda J and Anthonisen N R (2006). Inhaled corticosteroids and mortality in COPD. *Chest* 130: 640–646.

Morice A H and Wrench C (2000). The role of the asthma nurse in treatment compliance and self-management following hospital admission. *Respir Med* 95: 851–856

National Asthma Campaign (2001). Asthma statistics. http://www.asthma-uk.co.uk/asthma4. htm (accessed January 2008).

NICE (National Institute for Clinical Excellence) (2004). Chronic obstructive pulmonary disease: management of chronic obstructive pulmonary disease in adults in primary and secondary care. http://www.nice.org.uk/pdf/CG012_niceguideline.pdf (accessed 10 January 2007).

Newell K (2006). Concordance with asthma medication: the nurse's role. *Nurs Stand* 20: 31–33.

NHS Prodigy (2008). The primary care management of acute and chronic asthma in adult and children. http://www.cks.library.nhs.uk/asthma/about_this_topic (accessed January 2008).

Nishimura K, Koyama H, Ikeda A, Sugiura N, Kawakatsu K and Izumi T (1996). The additive effect of theophylline on a high-dose combination of inhaled salbutamol and ipratropium bromide in stable COPD. *Chest* 107: 718–723.

Rabe K F, Vermeire P A, Soriano J B and Maier W C (2000). Clinical management of asthma in 1999: the Asthma Insights and Reality in Europe (AIRE) study. *Eur Respir J* 16: 802–807.

Ram F S, Jardin J R, Atallah A, Castro A A, Mazzini R, Goldstein R, Lacasse Y and Cendon S (2005). Efficacy of theophylline in people with stable chronic obstructive pulmonary disease: a systematic review and meta-analysis. *Respir Med* 99: 135–144.

Roberts J (2002). The management of poorly controlled asthma. *Primary Health Care* 12: 43–49.

Settipane R J, Hagy G W and Settipane G A (1994). Long-term risk factors for developing asthma and allergic rhinitis: a 23–year follow-up study of college students. *Allergy Proc* 15: 21–25.

SIGN and BTS (Scottish Intercollegiate Guidelines Network and British Thoracic Society) (2007). British guideline on the management of asthma: a national clinical guideline. http://www.sign.ac.uk/pdf/sign63.pdf (accessed 10 December 2007).

Skoner D P (2000). Complications of allergic rhinitis. *J Allergy Clin Immunol* 105: 605–609.

Spergel J M and Paller A S (2003). Atopic dermatitis and the allergic march. *J Allergy Clin Immunol* 112 (6 suppl): S118–127.

Suissa S, Ernst P and Kezouh A (2002). Regular use of inhaled corticosteroids and the long term prevention of hospitalisation for asthma. *Thorax* 57: 880–884.

Thomas P, Pugsley J A and Stewart J H (1992). Theophylline and salbutamol improve pulmonary function in patients with irreversible chronic obstructive pulmonary disease. *Chest* 101: 160–165.

Tsukino M, Nishimura K, Ikeda A, Hajiro T, Koyama H and Izumi T (1998). Effects of theophylline and ipratropium bromide on exercise performance in patients with stable chronic obstructive pulmonary disease. *Thorax* 53: 269–273.

Vogelmeier C, D'Urzo A, Pauwels R, Merino J M, Jaspal M, Boutet S, Naya I and Price D (2005). Budesonide/formoterol maintenance and reliever therapy: an effective asthma treatment option? *Eur Respir J* 26: 819–828.

Wilts T J, Niewoehner D, Kim C, Kane R L, Linabery A, Tacklind J, MacDonald R and Rutks I (2005). Use of spirometry for case finding, diagnosis, and management of chronic obstructive pulmonary disease (COPD). Evidence report/Technology. Assessment No: 121. http://www.ncbi.nlm.nih.gov/books/bv.fcgi?rid=hstat1b.chapter.5 (accessed 10 January 2007).

# 10

# Prescribing in oncology

*Nicola Stoner*

---

**Key learning points:**

- Overview of the disease state
- Key issues for prescribing in this clinical area
- Overview of knowledge and skills for safe and effective prescribing
- Clinical case studies to demonstrate issues in non-medical prescribing.

---

## Pathophysiology, signs and symptoms, and prevalence

Oncology is the practice of treating tumours. A tumour is any abnormal swelling, and cancer is defined as any malignant tumour. A malignant tumour is one that invades and destroys the tissue in which it originates and can spread. Cancer is a disease of the cell cycle, which occurs through a multistep process. All cancers are caused through an accumulation of mutations within the DNA of a cell that in turn changes the genes that regulate cell growth and behaviour. This leads to a deregulation of cellular growth and cell division. For example, the tumour suppressor gene p53, which is located on chromosome 17, usually prevents cell division and is needed to initiate apoptosis. Any loss or alteration of the p53 gene can lead to a variety of tumours, including breast or colon cancer. The genetic damage causing cancers can either be inherited, caused by chemical carcinogens, viruses, lifestyle associations or by radiation. One in three of the population will be diagnosed with cancer in their lifetime, and one in four will die of cancer.

Tumours usually present as an abnormal swelling. Patients can also complain of fatigue, pain and weight loss. In order to diagnose the tumour, a fine needle biopsy, surgical biopsy and/or excision of the mass is taken to get a tissue sample that is analysed for its histology. Radiological imaging is also undertaken which can include an X-ray, ultrasound, magnetic resonance imaging (MRI), computed tomography (CT) or positron emission tomography (PET) scan. Tumour markers can also be used to diagnose, monitor response to treatment and give an indication of prognosis.

Tumours are classified according to the tissue of origin. The tumour is staged using a classification system that reflects the tumour burden and extent of the disease.

Cancer is treated with surgery, radiotherapy, cytotoxic chemotherapy, immunotherapy, endocrine therapy, and bone marrow or peripheral stem cell transplantation. The factors that affect the treatment decisions are histological diagnosis, the sensitivity of the disease to treatment, the stage of disease, patient performance status, patient choice and the aim of treatment. Treatment aims can include cure, prolongation of survival or palliation of symptoms. Adjuvant chemotherapy is given after surgery to improve survival by killing any micro-metastases. Neo-adjuvant chemotherapy is given prior to surgery to reduce the tumour burden and improve outcome. When deciding on the appropriate treatment for a patient, the clinician needs to decide on realistic goals of the treatment, assess the risk of the treatment against the potential benefit, consider the drugs that are available to treat that tumour type, and which line of treatment the patient is receiving.

A holistic approach needs to be taken when prescribing for cancer patients. Patients require support as they can often experience trauma following their diagnosis, suffer from emotional distress, fear, anxiety, anger, confusion, sense of loss, alienation, sadness and depression. This also has an effect on their family and friends, which needs to be taken into account. Cancer patients have to be counselled on the reasons for and benefits of taking their medication to aid compliance and concordance, as they may previously never have taken any medication.

## Knowledge and skills required for prescribing in oncology

The knowledge and skills required for prescribing in oncology include:

- understanding of the pathophysiology and presentation of the cancer
- monitoring of the cancer progression, e.g. tumour markers, radiological imaging, signs and symptoms, potential sites of metastases
- knowledge of chemotherapy treatment and its side-effects
- awareness of supportive care treatment requirements and their side-effects
- knowledge of local, network and national policies for chemotherapy and supportive treatment for cancer patients
- good communication skills
- ability to deal with terminally ill patients and their relatives
- understanding of the holistic care of the cancer patient

- awareness of non-drug and alternative treatments used for cancer and its symptoms
- experience of working in a multidisciplinary team treating oncology patients.

## General principles of prescribing in oncology

### Chemotherapy

The network chemotherapy protocol to be prescribed would normally be decided by the consultant oncologist following initial diagnosis and discussion at the local multidisciplinary team meeting. The non-medical prescriber must ensure they follow local prescribing policies and communicate well with the multidisciplinary team at all stages of the patient's care.

When prescribing in oncology, the prescriber must be aware of the patient diagnosis, prognosis, stage of disease and the planned outcome of the treatment, that is, is the treatment palliative, curative, adjuvant or neo-adjuvant. The patient's performance status and clinical condition also needs to be taken into account. The patient must have been informed and given written information about their chemotherapy treatment and its side-effects, and to have consented to receiving chemotherapy treatment. The patient must be monitored and assessed to ensure that the treatment is being effective, the side-effects are controlled and that the disease is not progressing. This is done using radiological imaging, tumour markers, good history taking and clinical examination.

Prescribed doses of cytotoxics are usually calculated on the basis of body surface area (BSA), which is measured in square metres ($m^2$). The dose is quoted as units (e.g. milligrams, grams, international units) per square metre. Patient surface area is calculated using a nomogram from patient height and weight measurements or using the following calculation:

$$\sqrt{\frac{(height\ (cm) \times weight\ (kg))}{3600}}$$

Obese patients have physiological changes that affect drug disposition, including increased blood volume, organ size and adipose tissue mass. Body surface area is often 'capped' at 2.0–2.2 $m^2$ in obese patients. The use of ideal body weight can be considered in these settings. However, the possibility of under-dosing needs to be considered in curative patients. There are some exceptions to doses being calculated on the basis of body surface area. Some chemotherapy drugs can be dosed according to patient weight, or using specific formulas. For example, carboplatin doses are based on the Calvert equation:

$$Dose\ (mg) = target\ AUC\ (GFR + 25)$$

where AUC is desired area under the plasma concentration curve (usually 5–7) and GFR is glomerular filtration rate.

Chemotherapy is usually administered at three-weekly intervals, and up to 8–12 cycles of treatment is usually prescribed. Some chemotherapy regimens are prescribed at weekly, two-weekly, or four-weekly intervals, and protocols must be checked to ensure chemotherapy regimens are prescribed at the appropriate intervals and duration.

Chemotherapy drugs must be given in appropriate doses, which are adapted to individual patients to allow the maximum probability of a desired therapeutic outcome with minimum toxicity. Cancer chemotherapy drugs often have a narrow therapeutic window between the dose that is effective and the dose that can be toxic, and inappropriate dose reduction can reduce chemotherapy efficacy. In organ dysfunction, it is essential to reduce chemotherapy doses to avoid serious or life-threatening toxicity. Chemotherapy should only be prescribed at the full protocol dose if the haematological and biochemical parameters are within the normal range.

Before prescribing chemotherapy, each patient must have their recent renal function, liver biochemistry tests, serum albumin and full blood count results checked. Biochemical parameters that need to be checked depend on the excreted route of the drug. Creatinine clearance should be monitored for renally cleared drugs, and liver function tests for those drugs metabolised hepatically. Myelosuppression is the most common and dangerous toxicity caused by chemotherapy, so all patients must have a blood count before each cycle of chemotherapy. Patients must only be administered chemotherapy if their white blood cell count (WBC) is $>3.0 \times 10^9/L$ (or neutrophils $>1.5 \times 10^9/L$) and platelets $>150 \times 10^9/L$. There may be exceptions to this in some local policies for patients with haematological malignancies, those undergoing intensive treatment with specialised support, or for patients with potentially curable tumours.

If the biochemical or haematological parameters are not within the normal range, then dose reduction or delay of subsequent doses needs to be considered. Doses are usually reduced by 20–25% initially. The size of the reduction depends on the nature and severity of the toxicity, taking into account whether the chemotherapy is palliative or curative in intent. Chemotherapy can be delayed by a few days to a week at a time if the haematological parameters have not returned to a safe range. Chemotherapy protocols should specify appropriate dose reductions or delays for specific regimens.

The adverse effects of chemotherapy must be considered when prescribing in oncology. The adverse effects can lead to dose reductions or delays in treatment, and can be both predictable and unpredictable. Each drug has its own spectrum of toxicity, and some examples will be given in the case studies below. General adverse effects to chemotherapy are seen in tissues where cells are continuously and rapidly dividing. Adverse effects of chemotherapy include myelosuppression, tumour lysis syndrome, electrolyte disturbances, skin reactions, anaphylaxis, mucositis, alopecia, nausea and vomiting, pulmonary toxicity, carcinogenicity, hepatotoxicity, cardiotoxicity, renal toxicity, neurotoxicity, extravasation and infertility.

## Supportive care

It is essential that supportive care is prescribed for oncology patients to counteract the toxicities of the chemotherapy, to manage the side-effects the patient is experiencing or to control the symptoms of their cancer. The general principles of prescribing for some of the main symptoms and side-effects experienced by oncology patients are detailed below.

### Chemotherapy-induced nausea and vomiting

Chemotherapy-induced nausea and vomiting is often the side-effect most feared by patients and may lead to patients refusing treatment. However, in practice it can be controlled in most cases by prescribing a combination of several antiemetic drugs. Only 20–30% of patients experience nausea and vomiting now that a wide variety of prophylactic antiemetics are available.

Chemotherapy drugs vary in the degree of nausea and vomiting they cause and are classified as mildly, moderately or highly emetic. Chemotherapy-induced nausea and vomiting is classified as acute (emesis during the first 24 hours after chemotherapy), delayed (emesis occurring more than 24 hours after chemotherapy) and anticipatory (conditioned vomiting response following inadequate antiemetic protection with previous cycles of chemotherapy). Patients at greater risk of chemotherapy-induced nausea and vomiting include women, those with a history of sickness in pregnancy, travel sickness, sickness after surgery, those who experienced sickness with previous chemotherapy, younger patients (less than 50 years of age) or patients with anxiety.

It is essential to prescribe appropriate antiemetics to prevent chemotherapy-induced nausea and vomiting as it can cause complications such as anorexia, malnutrition, dehydration, electrolyte and acid–base disturbances, and the development of anticipatory nausea and vomiting.

It is useful to inform patients of some non-drug measures to help prevent nausea and vomiting. These include avoiding factors that precipitate nausea such as the sight and smell of food, eating small and frequent meals, drinking flat fizzy drinks, eating or drinking items that contain ginger. Patients may want to explore the use of acupuncture or sea-bands.

When prescribing an antiemetic regimen one needs to consider the emetic risk of the chemotherapy regimen (degree, timing), the mechanism of action of the drugs available, the patient factors (drug history, medical history, previous response to antiemetics, predisposing factors), the effects of the drugs on gastric motility, the adverse effects of the antiemetics and cost effectiveness. If antiemetics are required, they should be prescribed regularly and prophylactically. It is essential to prescribe antiemetics to ensure optimal emetic control in the acute phase to prevent nausea and vomiting in the delayed phase.

Other causes of nausea and vomiting which need to be considered include radiotherapy, radio-sensitisers, infection, metabolic disorders, electrolyte disturbances, constipation, gastrointestinal obstruction, cachexia syndrome, metastases (brain, liver, bone), paraneoplasia or other emetic medications (e.g. opioids, antibiotics, antifungals). It is much easier to prevent nausea and vomiting than to treat it once it starts.

The route of administration prescribed needs to be considered, particularly for patients who may not be able to tolerate the oral route due to vomiting. If patients are unable to take oral antiemetics, consider prescribing them intravenously, subcutaneouosly, rectally or sublingually if they are available in those formulations. Antiemetics should be reviewed frequently and regularly.

The drugs that are prescribed for chemotherapy-induced nausea and vomiting include a $5HT_3$ receptor antagonist (e.g. ondansetron, granisetron), dexamethasone, metoclopramide, domperidone, cyclizine, levomepromazine and lorazepam. Local policies should be adhered to when prescribing antiemetics to prevent chemotherapy-induced nausea and vomiting. Considerations for prescribing these agents are noted below.

### $5HT_3$ receptor antagonists
These block $5HT_3$ receptors both centrally and in the gastrointestinal system involved in the pathophysiology of acute nausea and vomiting. They are prescribed for acute nausea and vomiting in moderately and highly emetic chemotherapy. Their main side-effects are constipation and headache. $5HT_3$ receptor antagonists are all equally efficacious and should be administered orally, and only for acute nausea and vomiting. There is only evidence for the use of $5HT_3$ receptor antagonists for an additional day in the delayed phase for cyclophosphamide and carboplatin-containing chemotherapy regimens.

### Dexamethasone
This has an unknown mechanism of action in chemotherapy-induced nausea and vomiting and acts synergistically with $5HT_3$ receptor antagonists. When given in combination, it increases the efficacy of other antiemetics by 20–30% for both acute and delayed nausea and vomiting. The main side-effects that patients need to be informed of include mood swings (mania and depression), increased appetite, heartburn and indigestion.

### Metoclopramide

This acts in the gastrointestinal tract as a prokinetic through $5HT_4$ agonist and dopamine-2 antagonist action, and centrally as a dopamine-2 antagonist. The main side-effects are restlessness and agitation, being unable to concentrate, stiff neck or jaw muscles and extrapyramidal side-effects.

### Domperidone

This acts in the gastrointestinal tract as a prokinetic as a dopamine-2 antagonist. It can be used instead of metoclopramide for patients experiencing extrapyramidal side-effects.

### Cyclizine

This acts centrally and has both antihistamine and antimuscarinic action. It is antikinetic, so should be avoided in combination with prokinetic antiemetics. Its main side-effect is sedation.

### Levomepromazine

This is a broad-spectrum antiemetic which is a dopamine-2 antagonist, antihistamine, antimuscarinic and $5HT_2$ receptor antagonist. It is useful for refractory emesis. Its main side-effect is sedation.

### Lorazepam

This is a benzodiazepine that acts on the cerebral cortex centrally. It is useful in anticipatory emesis. It causes sedation and amnesia. For pharmacist non-medical prescribers it is classified as a controlled drug, so can only be prescribed using a clinical management plan as a supplementary prescriber.

### Aprepitant

This is a neurokinin-1 receptor antagonist and should only be prescribed for acute nausea and vomiting for highly emetogenic cisplatin-based chemotherapy, as an adjunct to dexamethasone and a $5HT_3$ receptor antagonist to prevent acute and delayed nausea and vomiting.

### Mucositis

Patients who are on 5-fluorouracil, methotrexate, doxorubicin, bleomycin or capecitabine chemotherapy may present with mucositis. Their symptoms can include pain, tingling, dry mouth, ulceration and loss of taste. Patients must ensure they have good oral hygiene and use prophylactic saline mouthwashes. Treatment includes the use of antiseptic mouthwashes, anti-inflammatory mouthwashes, aspirin gargles, sucralfate suspension, mouth ulcer treatments and pain control.

### Diarrhoea

Diarrhoea can be caused by 5-fluorouracil, capecitabine and irinotecan. It can be managed by prescribing loperamide or codeine phosphate. An atropine premedication is prescribed with irinotecan to prevent cholinergic syndrome.

### Constipation

This can be caused by vinca alkaloid chemotherapy agents or by $5HT_3$ receptor antagonists. Laxatives can be prescribed according to the local policy.

### Palmar plantar syndrome

Palmar plantar syndrome can be caused by capecitabine, 5-fluorouracil and liposomal doxorubicin. The symptoms include redness, tingling, numbness, pain or swelling of the palms of the hands and/or soles of the feet. Pyridoxine 50–100 mg orally three times a day can be prescribed to treat this side-effect. Grade 2 or 3 symptoms may necessitate a chemotherapy dose reduction according to the local chemotherapy protocol.

### Renal toxicity

This can be caused by cisplatin, methotrexate, ifosfamide and cyclophosphamide. The patient's glomerular filtration rate (GFR) must be checked prior to chemotherapy. This can be calculated using the Cockroft–Gault equation in adults:

$$Creatinine\ clearance\ (mL/min) = \frac{F(140-age) \times weight\ (kg)}{Serum\ creatinine\ (\mu mol/L)}$$

where $F = 1.04$ in females and $1.23$ in males.

Alternatively, measuring creatinine clearance from a 24-hour urine collection or from an EDTA test in nuclear medicine is more accurate than the estimated calculation of GFR. Hydration schedules are prescribed with the chemotherapy to maintain a diuresis of $>100$ mL/hour. The plasma urea and creatinine must be monitored. Extra care must be taken with prescribing other nephrotoxic drugs such as furosemide.

### Electrolyte disturbances

Cisplatin is the main chemotherapy agent that can cause electrolyte disturbances due to damage in the renal tubules and collecting ducts. This can result in hypomagnesaemia, hypokalaemia, hypocalcaemia and hyponatraemia. Prophylactic potassium and magnesium are usually prescribed in the pre- and post-hydration bags administered with cisplatin.

## Prescribing issues from personal experience

Non-medical prescribers can prescribe both chemotherapy and supportive treatment, dependent on their competence. Chemotherapy is a potentially very toxic treatment and should only be prescribed by experienced and competent practitioners. Prescribers may want to consider prescribing chemotherapy as a supplementary prescriber initially, and once experienced in prescribing these drugs, to move on to prescribing them independently. Consideration should be given to using a flow sheet as an aide-mémoire for prescribing chemotherapy.

Prescribing protocols for chemotherapy and supportive care should be available in any unit where these treatments are prescribed. These should be followed at all times by non-medical prescribers. All prescribing should be evidence based and follow local formularies. Any variations to these protocols should be evidence based and documented, with the reasons why written in the patient's medical notes. There are times that there may be more than one way to approach a prescribing decision, and medical prescribers may dispute the prescription if they felt the other alternative could have been better. Neither prescriber is necessarily incorrect.

Good symptom control is essential for cancer patients, and improves their quality of life. Areas of supportive treatment where non-medical prescribers have a valuable contribution to patient care in oncology include antiemetics for chemotherapy-induced nausea and vomiting, laxatives, pain control, mouthcare, granulocyte-colony stimulating factors, and other supporting therapy required according to the chemotherapy protocols.

At the time of writing, pharmacists are unable to prescribe controlled drugs and nurses are only able to prescribe from a limited list of controlled drugs. As many cancer patients are taking pain relief classified as controlled drugs, non-medical prescribers need to ensure they can practice in accordance with the legislation. Consideration should be given to prescribing controlled drugs as a supplementary prescriber.

## Case studies

### Case study 1

A 46-year-old female patient presents to the inpatient chemotherapy pre-assessment clinic for cycle 1 of palliative treatment with gemcitabine ($1000$ mg/m$^2$ days 1 and 8) and cisplatin ($70$ mg/m$^2$ day 1) chemotherapy for bladder cancer. It is planned for her to have up to six cycles of chemotherapy. Her performance status is 0. Her height 165 cm, weight 78 kg, and surface area 1.86 m$^2$. She is on no medication and has no known drug allergies.

### 1 What antiemetics should be prescribed for this patient?

The antiemetics should be prescribed orally according to the local policy or the American Society of Clinical Oncology (ASCO) guidelines, for example:

- Dexamethasone tablets 8 mg twice a day for 2 days, then 4 mg twice a day for 3 days, then stop.
- Ondansetron 8 mg tablet 1 hour before chemotherapy and 12 hours later.
- Metoclopramide 10–20 mg four times a day starting day 1 and 8 of chemotherapy, regularly for 3–5 days then if needed.

**2 What counselling points should be covered with the patient about her medication?**

The patient is counselled on the possible side-effects of the chemotherapy, and given a patient information leaflet. The side-effects the patient may experience include acute and delayed nausea and vomiting (high emetic risk with cisplatin), a metallic taste in the mouth, flu-like syndrome, mucositis, diarrhoea, constipation, rash with pruritus, risk of nephrotoxicity, peripheral neuropathy, ototoxicity, fatigue and bone marrow depression (infection/bleeding/anaemia). The patient is informed that she will have a blood test to check that her blood count is back to normal the day before the next chemotherapy treatment. This blood test will also be used to monitor how well her kidneys are working following the treatment.

The patient is informed that she will receive anti-sickness medicines with her chemotherapy to prevent any nausea and vomiting. If she feels sick or are sick on the ward, she can ask for additional anti-sickness medicines. She is to receive three different anti-sickness medicines while she is an inpatient on the ward, and two anti-sickness medicines to take home after her overnight inpatient stay. The patient needs to be informed of the side-effects of the antiemetics, which are discussed above.

**3 The patient is worried about being sick with her chemotherapy, as she suffered from sickness in her two pregnancies, is travel sick and has been sick after surgery. How would the patient's concerns affect the antiemetic prescription?**

As this patient has several factors predisposing her to chemotherapy-induced nausea and vomiting, it is essential that additional antiemetics are prescribed during her inpatient stay. She could be prescribed lorazepam 1 mg at night orally as an inpatient and for 3 days at home, in addition to the antiemetics prescribed above. This combination works well, particularly for anxious patients. Lorazepam would need to be prescribed using a clinical management plan as a supplementary prescriber.

Alternatively, the patient could be prescribed levomepromazine 6.25–12.5 mg nightly instead of the night-time metoclopramide dose. Levomepromazine only needs to be administered once a day, and as it causes drowsiness it is best given at night.

**4. If the patient vomits on the ward, and is moderately nauseous for one week after chemotherapy, how could her antiemetics be adjusted?**

For the acute vomiting on the ward, lorazepam 1 mg could be prescribed regularly three times a day orally. Metoclopramide can be increased to 20 mg four times a day on discharge for 7 days. Alternatively metoclopramide could be replaced with cyclizine 50 mg three times a day or prochlorperazine 5–10 mg four times a day. Dexamethasone can be continued for longer at a reducing dose, for example an additional 2–4 days of dexamethasone 4 mg daily could be prescribed.

## Case study 2

The patient in case 1 returns to the inpatient chemotherapy pre-assessment clinic for cycle 4 of her gemcitabine and cisplatin chemotherapy. Her CT scan showed a response after three cycles of treatment, so it is planned for her to receive a total of six cycles of treatment. She presents with grade 2 fatigue, grade 1 alopecia, grade 0 stomatitis. She is constipated after chemotherapy. She has occasional tingling in her fingers and toes, but still manages to do her buttons up easily.

### Biochemistry results prior to cycle 4
- Sodium 136 mmol/L (135–145)
- Potassium 4.3 mmol/L (3.5–5.0)
- Urea 9.8 mmol/L (2.5–6.7)
- Creatinine 155 µmol/L (70–150)
- Bilirubin 5 µmol/L (3–17)
- Alanine aminotransferase (ALT) 12 iu/L (10–45)
- Alkaline phosphatase 150 iu/L (95–320)
- Gamma glutamyltranspeptidase (GGT) 18 iu/L (15–40)
- Phosphate 1.16 mmol/L (0.8–1.45)
- Magnesium 0.83 mmol/L (0.75–1.05)
- Lactate dehydrogenase (LDH) 200 iu/L (110–250)
- EDTA 46 mL/min.

### Haematology results
- Haemoglobin 12 g/dL (13–17)
- White cells 6.29 × $10^9$/L (4–11)
- Platelets 333 × $10^9$/L (150–400)
- Neutrophils 3.33 × $10^9$/L (2–7).

### 1 What are the prescribing issues with this chemotherapy regimen?

Gemcitabine and cisplatin chemotherapy is prescribed with 4 L of hydration fluid each day, so it is essential that fluid balance and patient weight is closely monitored. The hydration should be maintaining a urine output of 100 mL/h during and for up to 8 hours after cisplatin administration. Magnesium and potassium are added to the hydration bags to compensate for the losses of these electrolytes from the renal tubules. For inpatients, hydration is prescribed as 1 L normal saline over 4 hours prior to cisplatin administration, and 2 L normal saline over 8 hours post cisplatin infusion. For example 8 mmol magnesium sulphate and 20 mmol potassium chloride is added to each of these normal saline bags. Furosemide 20–40 mg orally or mannitol 10–20% injection 100–200 mL over 15–30 minutes respectively needs to be prescribed as required in case of fluid overload. This would normally be administered if the patient gained more than 1.5 kg during chemotherapy treatment or if urine output is less than 100 mL/h during intravenous fluid administration post cisplatin.

Note that patients on cisplatin regimens are at risk of increased nephrotoxicity if furosemide is added to the regimen.

It is essential that biochemistry and haematology results are checked on the day of chemotherapy administration, before the prescription is authorised. In practice, chemotherapy is often ordered in advance of the patient presenting at the clinic, however, the results must be checked before chemotherapy is released from the pharmacy and authorised for administration. The full blood count must be acceptable before chemotherapy is administered.

Biochemistry must be checked to assess renal function. Cisplatin is excreted renally and is nephrotoxic. If there is an abnormality in the biochemistry, dose reductions may be required. In this case, the patient's creatinine clearance is reduced to 46 mL/min according to the EDTA result. The cisplatin dose would have to be reduced by 50% with this creatinine clearance. British Oncology Pharmacy Association (BOPA) guidance states: GFR 50–60 mL/min 25% dose reduction, GFR 40–50 mL/min 50% dose reduction, omit cisplatin if GFR <40 mL/min.

The patient also has a raised creatinine and urea, which could be due to cisplatin-induced nephrotoxicity. The patient needs to be counselled on ensuring she keeps well hydrated while on cisplatin chemotherapy, as the high urea may indicate dehydration.

### 2 How should the patient's constipation be managed?

Senna two tablets at night for 3 days after discharge needs to be added to the discharge prescription for constipation. Other simple laxatives could be used instead of senna if preferred or according to local policy. For example, lactulose or sodium docusate. The most likely cause of the constipation is the $5HT_3$ receptor antagonist antiemetics.

## Case study 3

A 75-year-old male patient with testicular seminoma presents to the inpatient chemotherapy clinic prior to receiving cycle 3 of etoposide and cisplatin chemotherapy. The patient complained of heartburn. He has generalised pain which he attributes to his rheumatoid arthritis, which is relieved by paracetamol which he takes as required. Grade 1 fatigue and lethargy. Grade 2 alopecia. Performance status 1. Drug intolerances or allergies: aspirin causes stomach problems.

### Regular medication
- Ferrous sulphate 200 mg once daily orally
- Paracetamol tablets 1 g when required up to four times a day orally
- Lactulose 15 mL twice daily orally
- Ondansetron 8 mg twice daily starting 1 hour before chemotherapy for 2 days orally
- Dexamethasone 8 mg twice daily starting morning of chemotherapy for 3 days, then
- Dexamethasone 4 mg twice daily for 3 days orally then stop.
- Metoclopramide 10–20 mg orally four times daily starting day of chemotherapy, and for 3 days after chemotherapy regularly, then if needed
- Pegfilgrastim 6 mg subcutaneously 24 hours after chemotherapy.

### Chemotherapy
- Etoposide 166 mg/m$^2$ days 1, 2, 3
- Cisplatin 50 mg/m$^2$ days 1, 2
- Hydration bags: 1 L pre- and 2 L post-hydration with cisplatin – each hydration bag consists of 1 L sodium chloride 0.9% with 20 mmol KCl and 8 mmol MgSO$_4$ over 4 hours.

### Biochemistry results
- Sodium 135 mmol/L (135–145)
- Potassium 3.0 mmol/L (3.5–5.0)
- Urea 5.7 mmol/L (2.5–6.7)
- Creatinine 111 µmol/L (70–150)
- Bilirubin 4 µmol/L (3–17)
- ALT 16 iu/L (10–45)
- Alkaline phosphatase 319 iu/L (95–320)
- GGT 39 iu/L (15–40)
- Phosphate 1.12 mmol/L (0.8–1.45)
- Magnesium 0.81 mmol/L (0.75–1.05)

- LDH 208 iu/L (110–250)
- Calculated creatinine clearance 51.5 mL/min.

Haematology results
- Haemoglobin 8.6 g/dL (13–17)
- White cells 15.63 × $10^9$/L (4–11)
- Platelets 763 × $10^9$/L (150–400)
- Neutrophils 11.10 × $10^9$/L (2–7).

**1 What additional treatment should be prescribed for this treatment cycle?**

The patient has a low potassium result, which could have been induced by the cisplatin nephrotoxicity. An oral potassium supplement needs to be prescribed orally for 3 days, and then reviewed. Alternatively, additional potassium could be prescribed in the intravenous pre- and post-hydration bags.

**2 How should the patient's pain be managed?**

The patient was concerned that if he took his pain medication regularly, that his body would get used to it. Paracetamol was prescribed regularly for the patient, and he was counselled. The patient was advised that it was preferable to take pain relief regularly, rather than each time there was an episode of pain, and that his body would not get used to the painkiller.

**3 How should the patient's heartburn be treated?**

The patient should be prescribed an antacid such as Gaviscon, 15 mL four times daily orally after food regularly for his heartburn. If this is not sufficient after one month's treatment, then prescribing omeprazole 20 mg daily orally should be considered. The dexamethasone could be contributing to the patient's heartburn.

**4 Why is a granulocyte-colony stimulating factor prescribed with this treatment?**

Pegfilgrastim is a granulocyte-colony stimulating factor (G-CSF) and is prescribed to ensure that the patient can receive their treatment on time, as it is of curative intent. Pegfilgrastim is only prescribed prophylactically for patients who are at high risk of a neutropenic episode, who have had to have treatment delayed on a previous cycle due to low neutrophil count, or if patients have been admitted with a neutropenic episode following a previous cycle of chemotherapy. G-CSF stimulates the production of neutrophils, and may reduce the duration of neutropenia and incidence of febrile neutropenia. There is no evidence that it improves survival. It is prescribed as a single dose which is administered 24 hours after the last chemotherapy dose.

## Case study 4

A 54-year-old male patient presents to the inpatient chemotherapy pre-assessment clinic for cycle 2 of epirubicin, cisplatin and 5-fluorouracil for gastric cancer. He complains of grade 1 nausea, which is continuous. He also has mucositis grade 2 with a very painful cheek ulcer. He is finding it difficult to eat with such a sore mouth. He has had oral thrush starting day 3 after chemotherapy on cycles 1 and 2, which prevented him eating. His GP prescribed fluconazole 50 mg once daily for 7 days. He also complains of being very tired, and has started to become breathless on exertion.

### Chemotherapy
- Epirubicin 50 mg/m$^2$ by intravenous bolus injection day 1
- Cisplatin 60 mg/m$^2$ intravenous infusion over 4 hours day 1
- 5-Fluorouracil 4200 mg/m$^2$ over 3 weeks continuous intravenous infusion
- Hydration: 1 L pre- and 2 L post-hydration with cisplatin – each hydration bag consists of 1 L sodium chloride 9% with 20 mmol KCl and 8 mmol $MgSO_4$ over 4 hours.

### Drug history
- Salbutamol inhaler 2 puffs four times daily as required
- Senna 1 at night for 3 days after chemotherapy
- Paracetamol 1 g four times daily as required
- Cyclizine 50 mg three times daily continuously for nausea
- Fluconazole 50 mg once daily on days 3–10 of chemotherapy cycle.

### Antiemetics with chemotherapy
- Ondansetron 8 mg twice daily orally for 1 day
- Dexamethasone 8 mg twice daily orally for 3 doses, then 4 mg twice daily for 3 days
- Cyclizine 50 mg three times daily orally.

### Biochemistry results
- Sodium 141 mmol/L (135–145)
- Potassium 4.0 mmol/L (3.5–5.0)
- Urea 6.5 mmol/L (2.5–6.7)
- Creatinine 102 µmol/L (70–150)
- Bilirubin 15 µmol/L (3–17)
- ALT 23 iu/L (10–45)
- Alkaline phosphatase 192 iu/L (95–320)
- Phosphate 1.14 mmol/L (0.8–1.45)
- Magnesium 0.78 mmol/L (0.75–1.05)

- LDH 177 iu/L (110–250)
- Calculated creatinine clearance 54 mL/min.

### Haematology results
- Haemoglobin 10 g/dL (13–17)
- White cells $4.9 \times 10^9$/L (4–11)
- Platelets $197 \times 10^9$/L (150–400)
- Neutrophils $2.45 \times 10^9$/L (2–7).

### 1 What should be prescribed for the patient's mucositis?
The patient should be using a saline mouthwash regularly twice a day to try to minimise the mucositis. He has tried Difflam mouthwash 20 ml four times daily, but finds that it 'burns'. This could be because of the alcohol content. Aspirin soluble tablets 300–600 mg dissolved in water and gargled can be an effective painkiller in this situation. The aspirin can either be swallowed or spat out. In addition, the patient could take regular analgesia, for example, paracetamol soluble 1 g four times daily orally. If this is not adequate, low-dose morphine solution 5 mg four hourly can be used as a mouthwash and swallowed. Morphine would have to be prescribed using a clinical management plan as a supplementary prescriber.

Sucralfate suspension 1 g four times daily is effective when used as a mouthwash and swallowed before eating. In addition, there are several products available for mouth ulcers, including Adcortyl in Orabase, choline salicylate dental gel (Bonjela), to name a few.

### 2 Should any treatment be prescribed to prevent oral thrush for the next cycle?
The main issue for this patient is mouthcare. As the patient has regularly suffered from oral thrush in between cycles, an oral antifungal agent needs to be prescribed. For example fluconazole 50 mg daily orally to be taken days 3–10 of each cycle of chemotherapy.

### 3 What non-drug treatment needs to be prescribed for this patient?
The patient also has a low haemoglobin value with symptoms of fatigue and breathlessness on exertion, and needs to be cross-matched and given a blood transfusion.

### Case study 5

A 45-year-old patient presents at the outpatient colorectal clinic prior to his first cycle of adjuvant capecitabine for colorectal cancer. He has no previous medical history of note and has no known drug allergies. Height 180 cm, weight 85 kg, surface area 2 m². His biochemistry and haematology results are in the normal ranges.

**1 What dose of capecitabine should be prescribed?**
The patient is prescribed capecitabine 2500 mg/m² per day = 5000 mg/day = 2500 mg twice daily for 14 days, every 3 weeks.

**2 What information should be given to the patient about his chemotherapy?**
The patient is counselled on the possible side-effects of capecitabine chemotherapy. These include diarrhoea and abdominal pain, nausea, tiredness, reduced white blood cells, red blood cells and platelets, loss of appetite and taste changes.

**3 What supportive treatments should be prescribed and how should the patient be counselled?**
Loperamide must be prescribed orally, 2 mg after each loose stool when needed up to a maximum of eight capsules in 24 hours for possible diarrhoea or abdominal pain. The patient must be advised that if he has more than four bowel movements each day or diarrhoea at night that does not settle with loperamide after 2–3 days, to contact the oncology unit.

Metoclopramide is prescribed 10–20 mg up to four times daily orally when required for nausea. Alternatively, another antiemetic, such as cyclizine 50 mg three times a day, could be prescribed.

The patient is advised to use a saline mouthwash twice a day to prevent a sore mouth and mouth ulcers.

The patient is informed that the palms of the hands and/or soles of the feet can tingle, become numb, painful, swollen or red, and he must inform the oncology unit. He may also have dry or itchy skin, and a rash can appear. He is prescribed aqueous cream at least twice a day to be applied to both his hands and feet.

**4 If the patient complains that the palms of his hands and soles of his feet are red and dry with some pain that resolves before his next cycle of chemotherapy, what changes could be made to the patient's prescription?**
The patient could be prescribed pyridoxine 50 mg three times a day orally. If the palmar planter syndrome has resolved prior to the next cycle, there is no need for a capecitabine dose reduction. However, this should be monitored at each cycle.

The patient should be advised if the hands do not improve to contact the oncology unit, as the capecitabine dose may need to be interrupted for his hands to recover.

**5 What are the considerations for patients being prescribed oral chemotherapy?**
Patients must be able to tolerate the oral route, be educated on the recognition and management of side-effects, and counselled to ensure concordance and compliance. Patients are responsible for administration and need support

so that they know what to do if there are side-effects, for example if they vomit or miss a dose. Patients need to be educated on the name of the drug, its dose, and what the capsule or tablet looks like. They need to know when to take the drug and for how long, whether the drug needs to be taken after food, before food, with a large glass of water, 20 minutes after the antiemetic, etc. They also need to know where the drug should be stored, any precautions, and when to call the unit, doctor, nurse or pharmacist, and the contact details of who to call.

## Further reading

Allwood M, Stanley A and Wright P (eds) (2002). *The Cytotoxics Handbook*, 4th edn. Abingdon: Radcliffe Medical Press.

American Society of Clinical Oncology (2006). American Society of Clinical Oncology guidelines for antiemetics in oncology: Update 2006. http://www.asco.org/portal/site/ASCO/menuitem.c543a013502b2a89de912310320041a0/?vgnextoid=cf6f8c393c458010VgnVCM100000ed730ad1RCRD&vgnextfmt=default (accessed 24 November 2007).

Brighton D and Wood M (eds) (2005). *The Royal Marsden Hospital Handbook of Cancer Chemotherapy. A Guide for the Multidisciplinary Team.* Edinburgh: Elsevier Limited.

Calvert A H, Newell D R, Gumbrell L A, O'Reily S, Burnell M, Boxall R E, Siddik Z H, Judson I R, Gore M E and Wiltshaw E (1989). Carboplatin dosage: prospective evaluation of a simple formula based on renal function. *J Clin Oncol* 7: 1748–1756.

Cassidy J, Bissett, D and Spence R A J (eds) (2002). *Oxford Handbook of Oncology.* Oxford: Oxford University Press.

Douglas G, Nicol F and Robertson C (2005). *Macleod's Clinical Examination*, 11th edn. Edinburgh: Elsevier Churchill Livingstone.

Gabriel S and Daniels S (2003). Dosage adjustment for cytotoxics in hepatic impairment. The North London Cancer Network. http://www.bopawebsite.org/Members/Guidelines.asp (accessed 24 November 2007).

Gabriel S and Daniels S (2003). Dosage adjustment for cytotoxics in renal impairment. The North London Cancer Network. http://www.bopawebsite.org/Members/Guidelines.asp (accessed 24 November 2007).

National Institute of Clinical Excellence (2006). Colon cancer (adjuvant) – capecitabine and oxaliplatin. http://www.nice.org.uk/guidance/index.jsp?action=byID&o=11574 (accessed 24 November 2007).

Summerhayes M and Daniels S (2003). *Practical Chemotherapy: A Multidisciplinary Guide.* Abingdon: Radcliffe Medical Press Ltd.

# 11

# Prescribing in mental health

*Fabrizio Schifano*

---

**Key learning points:**

- Overview of the disease state
- Key issues for prescribing in this clinical area
- Overview of knowledge and skills for safe and effective prescribing
- Clinical case studies to demonstrate issues in non-medical prescribing.

---

## Introduction

With costs of the National Health Service (NHS) rising, the medicines bill is at about 11% of the total, despite a constant growth every year in the number of prescriptions issued (Association of the British Pharmaceutical Industry, 2007). On the other hand, medicines have made a significant contribution to the reduction in the use of hospital beds that has taken place over the past 30 years (Association of the British Pharmaceutical Industry, 2007). Most pharmaceutical/pharmacological research is carried out only in a few areas, including cancer, heart disease, stroke and disorders of the central nervous system (CNS). Costs of prescriptions dispensed in the UK related to CNS issues increased by 325% (from £510 million to £1658 million) during the period 1995–2003 and the number of CNS prescriptions dispensed (UK, 1994–2003) increased by more than 60% (from 94 million to 149 million). In parallel with increased number of CNS prescriptions, between 1970 and 2002 estimated savings due to reduced use of neurological and psychiatric hospital beds increased year-per-year from £43 million to £7734 million (Association of the British Pharmaceutical Industry, 2007).

Alongside the issue of prescription costs there is, of course, the cost of the prescribers themselves. Apparently GPs' salaries in the UK are currently the highest in Europe (Martin, 2007), so one could argue that the availability of non-medical prescription activities may be associated with a decrease in NHS costs. This might be achieved (National Pharmaceutical Association, 2005) through several possible routes:

- mean decreased administration costs for Primary Care Trusts (PCTs) compared with setting up and auditing minor ailment schemes
- GP time freed up to enable those who really need to see a doctor to do so
- opportunities to provide new and more cost-effective services for patients
- fewer calls to out-of-hours centres and decrease of indirect costs for private prescriptions.

In fact, although GPs can write private prescriptions for NHS patients, they still need to use an NHS appointment slot in order to obtain their own private prescription. Furthermore, with the introduction of pharmacists' independent prescribing, patients would be able to choose whether to see a GP or use a pharmacist, nurse or walk-in centre and may have faster access to NHS services. The many benefits of pharmacies include long opening hours and convenient locations close to where people live and work (National Pharmaceutical Association, 2005).

Although CNS medications and mental health issues account for a significant proportion of the issues related to NHS costs, there is still only little knowledge in terms of the impact that non-medical prescribing may have in mental health. This chapter therefore offers an overview of the very limited recent peer-reviewed literature available and comments on a few areas that may need further scientific debate.

## Pathophysiology of mental health disturbances

Psychiatric disorders are usually the result of a number of interacting/contributing factors. In fact, there may be genetics, social, environmental and psychological causes for mental illness.

Research suggests that some clients have inherited a genetic predisposition to clinical depression and that it is also likely to play a part in some cases of manic depression. Genetic predisposition is a contributing factor for some people who develop schizophrenia. In fact, the chances of developing that illness increase 10 times if the proband has a parent with schizophrenia. A genetic predisposition for some types of anxiety has been reported as well. People are more at risk of developing mental health problems if they have experienced certain traumatic events in the past, such as the loss of their parents during childhood, or abuse/neglect within the family. Stress may contribute to the development of mental health problems as well; as may a number of significant events or changes in life (e.g. having a baby, moving home, bereavement, losing a job, relationship break-up). On the other hand, there are specific mental health problems, such as depression, that can be associated with a number of physical conditions, including thyroid deficiency and pancreatic cancer.

## Prevalence of mental health disturbances

It is estimated that some 15–25% of people will suffer from a mental health problem at some point in their lives (Mental Health Foundation, 2008). Mental health problems are found in people of all ages, regions, countries and societies. It is estimated that approximately 450 million people worldwide have a mental health problem. Schizophrenia may affect roughly 1% of the adult population, but some 8–12% of the population typically experience depression in any given year. Depression is more common in women than men; 1 in 4 women will require treatment for depression at some time, compared with 1 in 10 men (Mental Health Foundation, 2008). Furthermore, women are twice as likely as men to experience anxiety, phobias or obsessive–compulsive syndromes. Conversely, men are more likely than women to have an alcohol or drug problem; almost three-quarters of people dependent on cannabis and 69% of those dependent on other illegal drugs are male. Depression affects 1 in 5 older people living in the community and 2 in 5 living in care homes. Dementia affects 5% of people over the age of 65 and 20% of those over 80 (Mental Health Foundation, 2008).

## Common signs and symptoms of mental health disturbances

Mental disorders have been defined as: 'health conditions that are character-ized by alterations in thinking, mood, or behaviour (or some combination thereof) associated with distress and/or impaired functioning' (MayoClinic.com, 2008). Mental health professionals typically define mental disorders by signs, symptoms and functional impairments. Signs, symptoms and func-tional impairments that mark specific mental illnesses are described in detail in the *Diagnostic and Statistical Manual of Mental Disorders* (DSM; American Psychiatric Association, 2000).

Signs and symptoms that should attract the attention of the health professional include (University of Dundee, 2008):

- poor appetite or compensatory overeating (eating disorders; depression)
- excessive tiredness (depression)
- poor concentration (depression)
- deterioration in self-care skills (e.g. personal hygiene) (depression)

- impaired motivation (depression)
- difficulty in remembering things (anxiety; depression; cognitive decline)
- problems in making decisions (anxiety; depression)
- loss of drive, energy and interest (depression)
- disturbed sleep pattern (stress; anxiety; depression)
- feeling low or miserable much of the time (depression)
- thoughts of suicide (depression)
- withdrawal from social events/contacts (depression)
- hearing or seeing things that others seem not to (schizophrenia; acute psychotic episode)
- increased irritability (personality disorder; hypomanic episode; depression)
- odd thinking (personality disorder; schizophrenia).

## A closer look: schizophrenia

Onset of schizophrenia typically occurs in late adolescence or early adulthood; the disease is often described in terms of 'positive' and 'negative' symptoms (NICE, 2002a, 2002b). Positive symptoms include delusions, auditory hallucinations and thought disorders and are typically regarded as manifestations of psychosis. Negative symptoms include flat, blunted or constricted affect and emotion, poverty of speech and lack of motivation. The client may show both disorganised speech (e.g. frequent derailment or incoherence) and behaviour. One or more major areas of functioning such as work, interpersonal relations or self-care, are markedly below the level achieved prior to the onset of schizophrenia. Typically, continuous signs of the disturbance persist for at least six months.

A diagnosis of schizophrenia is excluded if the symptoms are the direct result of a substance abuse or a general medical condition.

Diagnosis is based on the self-reported experiences of the patient, in combination with the signs identified. There are no reliable biological markers for schizophrenia, though studies suggest that genetics and neurobiology are important contributory factors. It is generally thought that a third of people might make a full recovery, about a third will show improvement, but not a full recovery, over time and a third of clients will remain ill. Women tend to show recovery rates higher than men. Acute and sudden onset of schizophrenia is associated with higher rates of recovery, while gradual onset is associated with lower rates.

## General principles of prescribing in schizophrenia

### Available treatment options for schizophrenia

Antipsychotics are classified into 'typical' and 'atypical' (Newcastle University, 2005; Gharabawi *et al.*, 2006).

* First-generation (typical) antipsychotics include: amisulpride; chlorpromazine; fluphenazine; haloperidol; promethazine; promazine; trifluoperazine.
* Second-generation (atypical) antipsychotics include: clozapine; olanzapine; quetiapine; risperidone; aripiprazole.

The typical therapeutic effect of antipsychotics is due to block of dopamine $D_2$ receptors, while the extrapyramidal symptoms (EPS) are due to dopamine antagonism in the basal ganglia (Newcastle University, 2005; Gharabawi *et al.*, 2006). Acute dystonias, often of jaw, neck or external ocular muscles may be observed in the first few days of treatment. Eventually, a parkinsonism (typically characterized by akinesia, rigidity and tremor) may manifest; this may respond to the use of antimuscarinic drugs (e.g. procyclidine, orphenadrine). A subjective restlessness of the legs often leading to pacing (akathisia) may appear within weeks of starting treatment but does not respond to antimuscarinics. The often irreversible tardive dyskinesia condition may appear after several months (Newcastle University, 2005; Gharabawi *et al.*, 2006); it is characterized by involuntary, choreiform movements mainly of mouth and face but sometimes also of limbs and trunk. Because dopamine is a prolactin inhibitory factor, dopamine blockade in the hypothalamus may also lead to hyperprolactinaemia with gynaecomastia, galactorrhoea and amenorrhoea.

Neuroleptic malignant syndrome is a rare but potentially fatal syndrome of rigidity, hyperpyrexia and confusion. Other side-effects include: blood dyscrasias, hepatitis, skin rashes and photosensitivity. Contraindications include: cardiovascular and cerebrovascular disease, parkinsonism, epilepsy, pregnancy and breast feeding, renal and hepatic impairment, prostatism, glaucoma. Interactions: increased effect of other hypotensives or sedatives (Newcastle University, 2005; Gharabawi *et al.*, 2006).

Typical antipsychotics may be usefully grouped according to their adverse effects profile (Newcastle University, 2005):

* Sedation +++; anticholinergic ++; extrapyramidal ++ (e.g. chlorpromazine)
* Sedation ++; anticholinergic +++; extrapyramidal + (e.g. thioridazine). The intrinsic anticholinergic activity of these drugs may limit their extrapyramidal effects but bears a higher risk of ECG changes.

- Sedation +; anticholinergic +; extrapyramidal +++ (e.g. haloperidol; flupenthixol decanoate; fluphenazine decanoate (decanoate formulations are used in depot preparations)).

Recently, several 'atypical', antipsychotics have entered the UK market. All these medication tend to be better tolerated than typical antipsychotics but may be more expensive as well. There is an ongoing debate about whether they should be prescribed 'first line' or reserved for patients who fail to respond or do not tolerate typical antipsychotics (Newcastle University, 2005; Gharabawi *et al.*, 2006).

Since clozapine is associated with potentially fatal agranulocytosis, it is only indicated in schizophrenia which has not responded to other antipsychotics. In addition, patients must have regular (initially weekly) blood counts performed before being prescribed the medication. Other adverse events include marked sedation, hypersalivation and anticholinergic effects, but EPS are less frequently seen than with typical antipsychotics. Risperidone, olanzapine and quetiapine show varying degrees of $5HT_2/D_2$ antagonism and are associated with weight gain but fewer EPS compared with typical antipsychotics. Risperidone can cause EPS, anticholinergic effects and hyperprolactinaemia at higher doses. Olanzapine is reasonably sedative; apart from its use in psychosis, a few data seem to emerge for the use of quetiapine in borderline personality conditions as well (Perrella *et al.*, 2007). Aripiprazole seems to have little effect on prolactin, glucose and lipid levels and QT interval in short- and long-term trials. Weight gain is similar to risperidone and less than olanzapine (UK Medicines Information, 2004).

The most important issue is to make sure that the client receives appropriate pharmacological treatment. One of the main problems in schizophrenia is given by lack of medication compliance. This is often due to lack of client collaboration, often explained by the intrinsic pathological characteristics of the disease itself. Both typical and atypical 'depot' antipsychotic formulations are available. Depot preparations are typically administered by intramuscular injection every 1–4 weeks. This may constitute a great advantage indeed in patients with poor compliance.

## Holistic approach in the treatment of mental health disturbances: the role of spirituality issues

Spirituality involves a dimension of human experience that psychiatrists are increasingly interested in, because of its potential benefits to mental health (Royal College of Psychiatrists, 2008). In healthcare, spirituality is identified with experiencing a deep-seated sense of meaning and purpose in life, together with a sense of belonging. It is about acceptance, integration and wholeness. From the spiritual perspective, a distinction can be made between cure, or relief of symptoms, and healing of the whole person (holistic approach). The universality of spirituality extends across creed and culture; at the same time spirituality is felt as unique to each and every person (Royal College of Psychiatrists, 2008). Patients have identified a number of benefits of good-quality spiritual care, including improved self-control, self-esteem and confidence; faster and easier recovery, achieved through both promoting the healthy grieving of loss and maximising personal potential; improved relationships – with both self and others; a new sense of meaning, resulting in reawakening of hope (Royal College of Psychiatrists, 2008).

## Knowledge and skills required for prescribing in mental health

The knowledge and skills required for prescribing in mental health include:

- understanding of the pathophysiology and presentation of all possible mental health problems
- knowledge of the prodromal signs of major mental health disturbances (e.g. depression; bipolar disorder; schizophrenia)
- awareness of antianxiety, antidepressant, antipsychotic and mood-stabilising treatments and side-effects
- (basic knowledge) of counselling principles
- excellent communication skills
- a non-judgemental, non-stigmatising and empathetic approach to the patient
- knowledge of local and national prescribing guidelines
- ability and willingness to deal with clients who may be chaotic, violent or suicidal
- large experience of working in different multidisciplinary teams treating the different mental health problems.

## Non-medical prescribing in mental health: an overview of the recent literature

McCann and Baker (2002) questioned whether community mental health nurse practitioners should have authority to prescribe medications. Their qualitative study used interviews and participant observation to collect data. The fieldwork was undertaken in the community, in regional and rural New South Wales, Australia and involved community mental health nurses. Respondents envisaged that prescribing authority would include most medications that are used to treat mental illness but exclude drugs that treat medical illness. Study participants also claimed that individual nurses who choose to forgo prescribing authority should not be coerced into undertaking this role.

Finley et al, (2003) pointed out that over the last 30 years clinical pharmacists have contributed to mental healthcare models in capacities ranging from educator to consultant to provider. In a systematic review, they evaluated the quantity and quality of medical literature examining the impact of pharmacists in mental health from 1972 to 2003. Although they identified approximately 35 publications describing the roles of clinical pharmacists in this regard, only 16 were of sufficient scientific rigour to allow evaluation and comparison. Nine of the studies examined the role of pharmacists in providing treatment recommendations and patient education, five featured pharmacists as providers, and the remaining two described the impact pharmacists have in delivering education to the psychiatric staff. Six of the 16 studies were prospective, but only three of these incorporated a randomisation procedure for patients or facilities. Collectively, the results of the 16 studies were positive, demonstrating improvements in outcomes, prescribing practices, patient satisfaction and resource use. Unfortunately, as pointed out by Finley *et al.* (2003), most of the investigations were small, and significant limitations in study design limited further comparison.

Jones (2006) aimed to explore perceptions held by nurses and psychiatrists towards the potential application of supplementary prescribing on acute psychiatric wards. Six focus groups were conducted with 19 nurses and 7 psychiatrists who worked on three wards located in North East Wales NHS Trust, Wrexham, UK. Two major themes were identified: first, ways in which patients could receive care and treatment through supplementary prescribing and in new forms of partnership and second, ways by which nurses and psychiatrists could be organised to deliver their care through a supplementary prescribing framework. Nurses and psychiatrists were generally positive about the advent of prescribing and offered positive views as to how patient care could be improved and a general willingness for nurses to adapt and work differently.

Hemingway and Davies (2005), from the UK, estimated that by 2005 at least some 4000 nurses had already completed the extended/supplementary prescribing course since its inception in 2003, with many more undertaking or planning to start the course. However, they emphasised that there is still a debate surrounding the issue of whether a generic course can meet the competency requirements of the differing nursing specialisms, such as mental health nursing. The authors carried out a study using a questionnaire survey distributed to an opportunistic sample of mental health nurses (MHNs) attending a national nurse prescribing conference and students who had completed the prescribing course. One hundred and fifty questionnaires were distributed with 89 returned, giving a response rate of 59%; 46 (52% of the sample) had completed or were undertaking the course, and 43 (48% of the sample) had not. The questionnaire aimed to elicit MHNs' experiences and perceptions of what they felt would help or hinder them developing as non-medical prescribers. Participating MHNs were asked the following question: 'What do you feel is the educational providers' role in facilitating a MHN becoming a nurse prescriber?' Although the course demands were perceived as a barrier by a number of candidates, most frequent (37; 34%) responses related to the need to concentrate the course content on 'mental health issues'. In this respect, a few suggestions were given by the students to include issues such as psychopharmacology, pharmacokinetics and pharmacodynamics of CNS drugs, overview of side-effects, legal and ethical guidelines, and concordance issues. Furthermore, according to respondents, a course should allow the nurse to facilitate 'theory and practice' (27 subjects; 24% of responses) but how this is delivered was questioned by the respondents.

Finally, Earles *et al.* (2006) commented on primary care clinical health psychology training as the appropriate mechanism for psychopharmacology education and practice. In the USA, the first class of psychologists graduated some 10 years ago with the Department of Defense Psychopharmacology Demonstration Project, which allowed these professional to prescribe within their area of expertise. Apparently, the programme received promising external reviews and audits. A number of professional schools and training institutions have implemented postdoctoral psychopharmacology training programmes and over 20 US states are actively pursuing legislative agendas.

## Non-medical prescribing policies in UK mental health trusts

(Notes taken from the Cambridgeshire and Peterborough Mental Health Partnership NHS Trust policy.)

The aim of the Cambridgeshire and Peterborough Mental Health Partnership NHS Trust policy (Gaskell, 2007) is to provide wider and faster access to medicines for service users, with more appropriate and flexible use of the workforce skills. A steering group has been locally established to lead on the development of non-medical prescribing within the Trust and to provide a support network for non-medical prescribers. Non-medical prescribing currently includes nurses and pharmacists working within the Trust.

According to the Trust policy, staff and line managers should use some guidance to determine suitability to undergo the non-medical prescribing course. Interested nurses should have a least 3 years' post registration clinical nursing experience, with one year preceding their application in the clinical area in which they wish to intend to prescribe. With respect to pharmacists, they should have at least 2 years' experience of professional practice in a mental health clinical environment. The Trust policy emphasises that non-medical prescribers will only prescribe medicines that are commonly used for mental health or substance misuse problems within their own service areas and that are on the Trust formulary. Furthermore, they are required to maintain a portfolio of their continuing professional development and should attend a minimum of three non-medical prescribing update sessions a year. These may be mental health trust-arranged sessions, PCT-arranged sessions, regional groups, university updates or national conferences. It is envisaged that the Trust will hold vicarious liability for non-medical prescribers where a number of criteria are met, including: the role of the non-medical prescriber is approved by the manager; the non-medical prescriber is working within the legal framework of the role and within Trust policies. Conversely, however, it is recommended that all non-medical prescribers affiliate to a trade union or professional organisation.

## Prescribing issues from personal experience

A few issues which clearly seem to require both further research and scientific input are briefly highlighted here.

Although the evidence at the moment is very limited, one might already identify the role of independent pharmacists prescribing in mental health. There may be a few areas where independent pharmacist prescribing in mental health would be appropriate, including:

- rationalising of patient medicines (e.g. altering doses, changing formulations, discontinuing unwanted or unnecessary medicines)
- involvement in lithium and clozapine monitoring clinics, to be able to alter doses without requesting a doctor's prescription
- acting on interventions arising from medicines use review (MUR), instead of unnecessary referral to the GP/consultant psychiatrist
- prescribing medicines (e.g. anxiolytics; antiepileptics) for patients in an emergency or out-of-hours.

It appears that the availability of non-medical prescribers throughout the UK is somewhat patchy. Some MH Trusts have anecdotally decided not to train any nurses or pharmacists to be prescribers. In other words, what seems to be a need identified from the Department of Health at a central level may be subject, at least at the present time, to different interpretations in different parts of the country. Conversely, it appears anecdotally that although some Trusts have facilitated the training of non-medical professionals in mental health, they have eventually restricted their capacity of prescribing due to budgetary limitation/cost-improving issues, resulting in a waste of training resources.

With regard to permanent learning, is 12 days provided by the prescribing course with the medical supervisor enough? The 12 days identified should be seen as a minimum, and the non-medical prescribers should be responsible for identifying their own learning needs and for planning their further education while in practice. According to the Sussex Partnership NHS Trust (2007), only those nurses and pharmacists who show evidence of ongoing mentoring in non-medical prescribing equivalent to at least 3.5 hours per month are eligible to be supplementary prescribers within the local Child and Adolescent Mental Health Services.

There is, at the moment, a blurring of roles between medical and non-medical prescribers. The situation might become even more complex if it is taken into account that in some English-speaking countries (e.g. USA) a number of clinical psychologists have been trained to prescribe within the mental health area. Furthermore, there is an ongoing discussion, in the USA, to allow them to prescribe in any area. Unfortunately, the blurring of roles might ultimately result in a blurring and confusing situation for the client.

## Case studies

### Case study 1: Depression resistant to treatment

A 27-year-old pharmacy student from the local university presents to her GP surgery with a number of symptoms which started just over three weeks ago, including tearfulness, irritability, social withdrawal, reduced sleep, lowered appetite (which has led to some weight loss), lack of libido, fatigue and marked anxiety. Along with a loss of interest and enjoyment in everyday life, feelings of guilt, worthlessness and deserved punishment, she complains of lowered self-esteem, loss of confidence, feelings of helplessness and suicidal ideation.

She is started with 20 mg fluoxetine tablets but, although she is compliant with her treatment, at all the clinical reviews carried out weekly over the eventual eight weeks the situation remains substantially unmodified. She is then reviewed by the local consultant psychiatrist and a prescription with clomipramine (up to 200 mg once daily) is started. Although the clinicians involved are fairly confident about the diagnosis (depressive episode) and the medication compliance levels, the clinical situation after eight more weeks of treatment is still unsatisfactory.

#### 1 What is the prevalence of depression?
The estimated point prevalence for major depression among 16- to 65-year olds in the UK is 2% but, if the less specific and broader category of 'mixed

depression and anxiety' is included, these figures rise dramatically to 10% (NICE, 2004a). Prevalence rates are greatly influenced by gender, age and marital status. Female preponderance is increased during adulthood, but after the age of 55 the sex ratio actually reverses.

## 2 What are the theoretical explanations for depression?

Theoretical explanations for depression aetiology include genetic, biochemical and endocrine, psychological, and social. Some physical illnesses do increase the risk of depression, including diabetes, cardiac disease, hyperthyroidism, hypothyroidism and Cushing's syndrome. A family history of depressive illness accounts for around 39% of the variance of depression in both sexes. Some episodes of depression occur in the absence of a stressful event, and conversely many such events are not followed by a depressive disorder (NICE, 2004a). Although it is generally thought that depression is usually a time-limited disorder lasting up to six months with complete recovery afterwards, it seems that after 2 years 40% of clients are still depressed. At least 50% of people following their first episode of major depression will go on to have at least one more episode (NICE, 2004a).

## 3 What are the pharmacological treatments and side-effects?

The mode of action of antidepressants is likely to be associated with their ability to block the synaptic reuptake of monoamines, including noradrenaline (NA), 5-hydroxytryptymine (5HT) and dopamine (DA). Conversely, the side-effects resulting from their ability to influence anticholinergic, histaminergic and other receptor systems may reduce their acceptability. Moreover, overdose with tricyclic antidepressants (TCAs) carries a high mortality and morbidity, which is particularly problematic in the treatment of people with suicidal intentions. In response to the side-effect profile and the toxicity of TCAs in overdose, new classes of antidepressants have been developed, including the specific serotonin reuptake inhibitors (SSRIs) such as fluoxetine; drugs chemically related to, but different from, the TCAs, such as trazodone; and a range of other chemically unrelated antidepressants including mirtazapine.

Other drugs used either alone or in combination with antidepressants include lithium salts and the antipsychotics, although the use of these drugs is usually reserved for people with severe, psychotic or chronic depressions, or as prophylactics.

## 4 What is treatment-resistant depression?

Some people with depression do not respond well to initial treatment. Treatment-resistant depression is defined as that which fails to respond to two or more antidepressants given sequentially at an adequate dose for an adequate time. Patients whose depression is treatment resistant may benefit from psychological interventions. For chronically depressed patients, the combination of pharmacological and psychological treatment may be particularly effective. For patients whose depression is treatment-resistant, the combination of antidepressant medication with cognitive behavioural therapy should be considered (NICE, 2004a). A trial of lithium augmentation should be considered for patients whose depression has failed to respond to several antidepressants. Venlafaxine should be considered for patients whose depression has failed to respond to two adequate trials of other antidepressants. For patients prescribed venlafaxine, consideration should be given to monitoring of cardiac function. Regular monitoring of blood pressure should be undertaken, particularly for those on higher doses.

## Case study 2: Bipolar disorder

Mr AB is a 35-year-old painter and decorator who presents to the local pharmacy with severe insomnia, irritability, aggressiveness, elated mood, disinhibited behaviour and excessive spending; furthermore, his partner reports of unusual sexual demands. His symptoms started 5 days ago; there is a previous history of three manic and four depressive episodes over the last 4 years. Odd binges with both cocaine and alcohol over the last 6 years are reported; last binge occurred two weeks ago. No previous medical history is given; up to a few months ago he was on long-term treatment with olanzapine tablets 10 mg once daily. Relevant test results do not identify any pathological issues and the diagnosis of manic episode, bipolar disorder, is given.

### 1 What is bipolar disorder?
To achieve a diagnosis of bipolar disorder in adults, most diagnostic systems require at least two episodes (one of which must be mania or hypomania) in which the person's mood and activity levels are significantly disturbed. The disturbance consists of either an elevation of mood and increased energy and activity (mania or hypomania), or a lowering of mood (depression). Manic episodes usually begin abruptly and are characterised by periods of over-active, disinhibited behaviour lasting at least 4 days. Drug and/or alcohol misuse may induce manic-like symptoms. Acute manic symptoms may be due to underlying organic conditions, such as hypothyroidism, cerebrovascular insults and other neurological disorders (for example, dementia), particularly in people with late-onset bipolar disorder (older than 40 years).

### 2 What are the pharmacological treatment options?
The following drugs have UK marketing authorisation for use in bipolar disorder (NICE 2006):

- for treatment of mania – lithium, olanzapine, quetiapine, risperidone, and valproic acid (as valproate semisodium)

- for prophylaxis – lithium and olanzapine
- for prophylaxis of bipolar disorder unresponsive to lithium – carbamazepine.

Lithium, olanzapine or valproate should be considered for long-term treatment of bipolar disorder. The choice should depend on:

- response to previous treatments
- the relative risk, and known precipitants, of manic versus depressive relapse
- physical risk factors, particularly renal disease, obesity and diabetes
- the patient's preference and history of adherence
- gender (valproate should not be prescribed for women of child-bearing potential).

Long-term drug treatment should normally continue for at least 2 years after an accurately diagnosed episode of bipolar disorder, and up to 5 years if the person has risk factors for relapse, such as a history of frequent relapses or severe psychotic episodes. Whilst olanzapine efficacy in schizophrenia might be mediated through a combination of both dopamine and serotonin type 2 ($5HT_2$) antagonism, its mechanism of action in the treatment of acute manic episodes is somewhat unknown. Although valproate's mechanism of action has not yet been established, the drug's anticonvulsant activity may be related to increased brain concentrations of gamma-aminobutyric acid (GABA). Valproic acid may produce teratogenicity; and the incidence of neural tube defects in the fetus may be increased when mothers are receiving valproic acid during the first trimester of pregnancy.

People with bipolar disorder should have periodic physical health reviews, to ensure that the following are assessed:

- lipid levels, including cholesterol, in all patients over 40 even if there is no other indication of risk
- plasma glucose levels
- weight
- smoking status and alcohol use
- blood pressure
- renal and thyroid function.

Healthcare professionals should discuss with patients the risk of weight gain, and be aware of the possibility of worsening existing diabetes, malignant neuroleptic syndrome and diabetic ketoacidosis with the use of antipsychotic medication.

**3 What are the essential counselling points regarding drug therapy assuming the patient is prescribed with lithium carbonate on a long-term basis?**

Before lithium is started, both height and weight should be measured and the following should be arranged: tests for urea and electrolytes, serum creatinine, thyroid function, ECG for patients with cardiovascular disease or risk factors for it, and full blood count. Thyroid and renal function tests should be arranged every six months, or more often if there is evidence of impaired renal function. Patients are to be informed that they should take lithium for at least six months to establish its effectiveness as a long-term treatment. Serum lithium levels should be checked one week after starting and one week after every dose change, and until levels are stable. The aim should be to maintain serum lithium levels between 0.4 and 0.8–1.0 mmol/L, depending on a number of clinical parameters. Contraception and the risks of pregnancy should be discussed with all women of child-bearing potential, regardless of whether they are planning a pregnancy.

Symptoms of neurotoxicity, including paraesthesia, ataxia, tremor and cognitive impairment, which can occur at therapeutic levels, should be regularly monitored. Patients taking lithium should be advised to seek medical attention if they develop diarrhoea and/or vomiting. They should ensure they maintain their fluid intake, particularly after sweating. Lithium should be stopped gradually over at least four weeks, and preferably over a period of up to three months, particularly if the patient has a history of manic relapse.

## Case study 3: Panic disorder with agoraphobia

FS, a 51-year-old academic, presents to his local surgery because of recurrence of unexpected panic attacks followed by two months of persistent concern about having another panic attack, worry about the possible implications or consequences of the panic attacks, and a significant behavioural change related to the attacks. He reports as well that in certain situations (like speaking in public, or going out for dinner with colleagues) he fears that he is 'going crazy' or losing control. FS fears that these panic attacks indicate the presence of an undiagnosed, life-threatening illness (such as cardiac disease). After a few reviews carried out by both the local GP and the cardiologist, it is confirmed that the patient's panic attacks are not due to the direct physiological effects of a substance or general medical condition, but FS remains frightened and unconvinced despite repeated medical testing and reassurance.

**1 What is the essential feature of panic disorder?**
The essential feature of panic disorder with agoraphobia is anxiety about being in places or situations from which escape might be difficult (or

embarrassing) or in which help may not be available in the event of having a panic attack (NICE, 2004b). This anxiety is said to typically lead to a pervasive avoidance of a variety of situations that may include: being alone outside the home or being home alone; being in a crowd of people; travelling by car, bus or place, or being on a bridge or in a lift. Transient tachycardia and moderate elevation of systolic blood pressure may occur during some panic attacks.

### 2 What are the pharmacological treatments options?

Unless otherwise indicated, an SSRI licensed for panic disorder should be offered. If an SSRI is not suitable or there is no improvement after a 12-week course and if a further medication is appropriate, imipramine or clomipramine may be considered. If the patient is showing improvement on treatment with an antidepressant, the medication should be continued for at least six months after the optimal dose is reached, after which the dose can be tapered. All patients prescribed antidepressants should be informed that, although the drugs are not associated with tolerance and craving, discontinuation/withdrawal symptoms may occur on stopping or missing doses or, occasionally, on reducing the dose of the drug. The most commonly experienced discontinuation/withdrawal symptoms are dizziness, numbness and tingling, gastrointestinal disturbances (particularly nausea and vomiting), headache, sweating, anxiety and sleep disturbances. Benzodiazepines are associated with a less good outcome in the long term and should not be prescribed for the treatment of individuals with panic disorder.

### Case study 4: Benzodiazepine dependence

A 39-year-old nurse has been taking lorazepam tablets 1.5 mg once daily for at least the last 10 years. She was initially started with lorazepam tablets 2.5 mg once daily some 15 years ago but she gradually increased the dosage over the following years. Both her GP and the local pharmacist have informed her that the situation needs to be addressed appropriately. She has tried unsuccessfully on a number of occasions to titrate down and stop the dosage over a period of few days/weeks. However, on all these occasions a number of signs and symptoms, including anxiety, restlessness, muscle aches, intolerance to sound and lights, insomnia and depression have appeared and, for this reason, she has lately resorted to a few rogue web sites to purchase further lorazepam tablets.

### 1 How is the benzodiazepine receptor structured? Can you expand on the pharmacodynamics of benzodiazepines?

Benzodiazepine receptors are associated with GABA chloride channel complex ($GABA_A$ receptor). Benzodiazepine receptor is a modulating unit, modifying the response to GABA. Agonists enhance submaximal responses to GABA (cannot enhance maximal responses), but benzodiazepines have no direct action on the chloride channel. Stimulation of BZ1 receptor results in hypnotic effects while BZ2 receptors mediate anticonvulsant effects. Increasing doses of benzodiazepines increase receptor occupancy and produce a progressive spectrum of effect from anxiolysis and anticonvulsant effects to amnesia, sedation and eventually hypnosis and anaesthesia.

Benzodiazepines are remarkably safe if taken alone and rapid reversal of sedation with the receptor antagonist flumazenil is rarely necessary or cost-effective. Even massive overdoses, if taken without other CNS depressants, are almost never fatal. This is because the opening up of the chloride ion channels depends on the availability of GABA, whose interaction with the receptor is facilitated by benzodiazepines liaising with their GABA receptor portion. This is different from what happens with barbiturates and alcohol, which interact with the chloride ion channels directly. As a consequence, high dosages of these compounds may facilitate a massive increase of chloride ions in the CNS cells, thus determining a generalised depression of CNS functions.

### 2 What is the typical duration of a benzodiazepine treatment?

Benzodiazepines are usually required for only short periods of treatment; the vast majority of actual prescription of these drugs lasts for only a few weeks. However, some disorders for which benzodiazepines are indicated are recurrent or chronic.

### 3 Can you better explain the epidemiological and clinical pharmacological issues related to both benzodiazepine misuse and benzodiazepine withdrawal syndrome?

Consumption of prescribed medications is higher in certain workplace environments (for a review, see Schifano, 2006), including the health sector. Findings suggest that it is unlikely that most use of benzodiazepines in patient populations is associated with a significant risk of abuse. It has been suggested that the onset of withdrawal might be more rapid and the intensity of withdrawal might be greater following discontinuation of short-acting benzodiazepines than after discontinuation of long-acting compounds. Most studies of therapeutic-dose dependence examined the effects of discontinuation in patients who had used the drugs for relatively long periods. However, withdrawal can be observed even after relatively brief periods of use (e.g. two weeks). Other factors that have been considered as possible determinants of the development of physiological dependence have included duration of drug action, magnitude of dose, patients' prior drug use, age and personality traits.

Upon abrupt discontinuation of benzodiazepine treatment, dependent patients are likely to experience increased anxiety and/or insomnia (the 'rebound syndrome'). In fact, the symptoms of anxiety/sleep disturbances for which these compounds were originally prescribed may well reappear. On the other hand, the proper benzodiazepine 'withdrawal syndrome' is character-ized by further signs and symptoms, including panic attacks, 'flu-like' syndrome, alterations in taste and smell sensations, tremor, restlessness, gastrointestinal distress, sweating, tachycardia and mild systolic hypertension (Schifano and Magni, 1989). In severe withdrawal states, hallucinations, seizures and deaths have been reported.

The syndrome and associated discomfort are usually, but not always, mild, reaching peak severity in 2–20 days and abating within four weeks after discontinuation. Clinical authorities have long recommended that use should be interrupted by occasional 'drug holidays', which would permit reassessment of the need to continue treatment and might also reduce the risk of dependence development.

**4 Which is the clinical approach to be taken into consideration when discontinuing a long-term benzodiazepine treatment?**
The maximum speed that can be reached is 10% of the previous daily dose (e.g. 100 mg; 90 mg; 81 mg; 73 mg, etc.). If dosages are higher than 30 mg of diazepam, reduction should be kept at 5–10 mg/month. While reducing, counselling, support groups and relaxation techniques can be helpful (Schifano and Magni, 1989).

### Case study 5: Cardiovascular effects of atypical antipsychotic drugs

A 48-years old client was diagnosed with schizophrenia some six months ago by the local consultant psychiatrist, and at that time initiated with olanzapine 20 mg once daily. Since then, the client had been regularly reviewed by the non-medical, supplementary prescriber (a mental health nurse). With this medication, the psychiatric situation achieved a satisfactory level of stabiliza-tion and for this reason no further review with the consultant psychiatrist was organised. After six months, the client started complaining of a few cardiovascular disturbances, including arrhythmic and syncopal events, which were then correctly interpreted by a cardiologist from whom his family sought private advice as a result of a drug-induced QT prolongation (Crumb et al., 2006).

1 In taking into account the above case scenario:
- Can you comment on the training respectively given to general/medical and mental health nurses?
- Are the mental health nurses trained well enough to interpret and understand the clinical pictures such as those here described and the ECG results?

- Can you comment on both the length and the topics that should be covered during the non-medical prescribing training?

This probably highlights a somewhat paradoxical situation. On one hand, a general nurse might be in a better position in terms of being able to interpret both the origin of the symptoms described and the ECG than a mental health nurse. Conversely, mental health nurses are clearly better trained to understand and interpret the complex psychiatric situation of their own clients. Issues arising from the case scenario are in line with the main issue identified in the present review (e.g. the need to organise the generic course content relevant to all the students on the prescribing course). It could be argued that all specialist non-medical prescribers would prefer a course designed to meet their own agenda, and this could be clearly true for non-medical prescribers in mental health as well. On the other hand, Hemingway and Davies (2005) suggest that to develop a course purely to meet the needs of certain specialisms could hinder appreciation of other professionals' role and in turn this could lead to fragmented patient care.

Furthermore, at the end of the course, non-medical prescribers will be technically allowed to prescribe from the whole of the formulary, although they are advised to prescribe within their own specialist area only. For example, it is unrealistic to believe that non-medical prescribers in mental health would not ever assess the needs of patients who are taking antibiotics. Knowledge of antibiotics may be considered most useful, considering the possible side-effects and interactions of most psychoactive compounds.

According to Hemingway and Davies (2005), courses need to be designed to meet global prescribing needs, and when considering inter-professional learning this would appear to be more appropriate. It may be suggested here that non-medical prescribers may need training not only in pharmacology, but also in medication management, diagnostics skills, as well as legal and professional accountability. Some non-medical prescribers might be in favour of a longer training prior to graduation to be allowed to prescribe (Hemingway and Davies, 2005).

One could argue that at least six months might be required for a generic teaching given to all non-medical professionals attending the course, to reserve the further semester to the different specialities. From this point of view, mental health professionals should be specifically trained, and thoroughly examined, in basic and clinical neuropsychopharmacological issues. It is strongly suggested here that all non-medical professionals, including pharmacists, should be extensively trained (and thoroughly examined) at both under-graduate and postgraduate level in both clinical and clinical pharmacological issues, given the likely increasing role of non-medical prescribers in future decades.

# References

American Psychiatric Association (2000). Diagnostic and Statistical Manual of Mental Disorders, Fourth Edition, Text Revision (DSM-IV-TR). Arlington VA: American Psychiatric Association.

Association of the British Pharmaceutical Industry (2007). Facts & statistics from the pharmaceutical industry. http://www.abpi.org.uk/statistics (accessed 24 October 2007).

Crumb W J Jr, Ekins S, Sarazan R D, Wikel J H, Wrighton S A, Carlson C and Beasley C M Jr. (2006). Effects of antipsychotic drugs on I(to), I(Na), I(sus), I(K1), and hERG: QT prolongation, structure activity relationship, and network analysis. *Pharm Res* 23: 1133–1143.

Earles J E, James L C and Folen R A (2006). Prescribing non-psychopharmacological agents: a new potential role for psychologists in primary care settings and specialty clinics. *J Clin Psychol* 62: 1213–1220.

Finley P R, Crismon M L and Rush A J (2003). Evaluating the impact of pharmacists in mental health: a systematic review. *Pharmacotherapy* 23: 1634–1644.

Gaskell C (2007). Non-medical Prescribing Policy. Cambridgeshire and Peterborough Mental Health Partnership NHS Trust, April 2007. http://www.cambsmh.nhs.uk/documents/Clinical/Non_medical_prescribing.pdf?preventCache=13%2F06%2F2007+12%3A31 (accessed 25 October 2007).

Gharabawi G M, Greenspan A, Rupnow M F, Kosik-Gonzalez C, Bossie C A, Zhu Y, Kalali A H, Awad A G (2006). Reduction in psychotic symptoms as a predictor of patient satisfaction with antipsychotic medication in schizophrenia: data from a randomized double-blind trial. *BMC Psychiatry* 61: 45.

Hemingway S and Davies J (2005). Non-medical prescribing education provision: how do we meet the needs of the diverse nursing specialisms? *Nurse Prescriber* 21 April, 2(4). http://www.nurse-prescriber.co.uk (accessed 24 October 2007).

Jones A (2006). Supplementary prescribing: potential ways to reform hospital psychiatric care. *J Psychiatr Ment Health Nurs* 13: 132–138

Martin D (2007). Highly paid British GPs are happier with their salary than any European counterpart. *The Daily Mail*, 25th October 2007. http://www.dailymail.co.uk/pages/live/articles/news/news.html?in_article_id=489579&in_page_id=1770 (accessed 26 October 2007).

MayoClinic.com (2008). Mental health: what's normal, what's not. http://www.mayoclinic.com/health/mental-health/MH00042 (accessed 11 May 2008).

McCann T V and Baker H (2002). Community mental health nurses and authority to prescribe medications: the way forward? *J Psychiatr Ment Health Nurs* 9: 175–182.

Mental Health Foundation (2008). Statistics on mental health. http://www.mentalhealth.org.uk/information/mental-health-overview/statistics/#howmany (accessed 11 May 2008).

National Pharmaceutical Association (2005). Final response to the MHRA consultation on proposals to introduce independent prescribing by pharmacists, MLX 321. May 2005. http://www.epolitix.com/NR/rdonlyres/048437E6-0A8A-42B6-A4A6-41889EE03A23/0/IndependentprescribingMLX321responseMay05.pdf (accessed 25 October 2007).

Newcastle University School of Neurology, Neurobiology & Psychiatry, Faculty of Medical Sciences (2005). Medical student teaching resource. Antipsychotics. http://www.ncl.ac.uk/nnp/teaching/management/drugrx/antpsych.html (accessed 2 April 2007).

NICE (National Institute for Clinical Excellence) (2002a). National Collaborating Centre for Mental Health. Schizophrenia: core interventions in the treatment and management of schizophrenia in primary and secondary care. London: National Institute for Clinical Excellence, 2002.

NICE (2002b). Treating and managing schizophrenia (core interventions). Understanding NICE guidance – information for people with schizophrenia, their advocates and carers, and the public. http://www.nice.org.uk (accessed 2 April 2007).

NICE (2004a) National clinical practice guideline number 23. Depression: management of depression in primary and secondary care. http://www.guideline.gov/summary/summary.aspx?doc_id=62281.

NICE (2004b). Clinical guidelines for the management of anxiety. Management of anxiety (panic disorder, with or without agoraphobia, and generalised anxiety disorder) in adults in primary, secondary and community care. http://www.nice.org.uk/CG221.

NICE (2006). Clinical guideline 38. Bipolar disorder: the management of bipolar disorder in adults, children and adolescents, in primary and secondary care, July 2006. http://www.nice.org.uk/CG038.

Perrella C, Carrus D, Costa E and Schifano F (2007). Quetiapine for the treatment of border-line personality disorder: an open label study. *Progr Neuropsychopharmacol Biol Psychiatry* 31: 158–163.

Royal College of Psychiatrists (2008). Spirituality and mental health. http://www.rcpsych.ac.uk/mentalhealthinformation/therapies/spiritualityandmentalhealth.aspx (accessed 11 May 2008).

Schifano F (2006). Substance misuse in the workplace. In: Ghodse A H (ed.). *Addiction at Work: Tackling Drug Use and Misuse in the Workplace.* London: Gower Publishing Ltd.

Schifano F and Magni G (1989). Panic attacks and major depression after discontinuation of long-term diazepam abuse. *Drug Intelligence and Clinical Pharmacy. Ann Pharmacother* 23: 989–990.

Sussex Partnership NHS Trust (2007). Children and Adolescent Mental Health Services. Protocol to support supplementary prescribing, April 2007.

UK Medicines Information (2004). Aripiprazole. http://www.ukmi.nhs.uk/NewMaterial/html/docs/AripiprazoleNMP0604.pdf (accessed 2 April 2007).

University of Dundee (2008). Mental health problems. http://www.dundee.ac.uk/healthservice/info_content/MentalHealthProblems.htm (accessed 11 May 2008).

# Index